Aids to Paediatrics for Undergraduates

# Aids to Paediatrics for Undergraduates

**Alex Habel**
MB ChB MRCP (UK)
Consultant Paediatrician,
West Middlesex Hospital,
Isleworth

SECOND EDITION

CHURCHILL LIVINGSTONE
EDINBURGH  LONDON  MADRID  MELBOURNE  NEW YORK  AND
TOKYO  1995

CHURCHILL LIVINGSTONE
Medical Division of Pearson Professional Limited

Distributed in the United States of America by Churchill Livingstone
Inc., 650 Avenue of the Americas, New York, N.Y. 10011, and by
associated companies, branches and representatives throughout
the world.

First edition 1987
Second edition 1995

ISBN  0-443-05206-9

British Library Cataloguing in Publication Data
A catalogue record for this book is available from the British
Library.

Library of Congress Cataloging in Publication Data
A catalog record for this book is available from the
Library of Congress.

The
publisher's
policy is to use
paper manufactured
from sustainable forests

Produced by Longman Singapore Publishers (Pte) Ltd
Printed in Singapore

# Preface

A systematic approach to problems, sifting the symptoms and signs gleaned at the bedside, is the hallmark of the well prepared candidate. My aim is to make that process easier, with what I hope is the correct balance for undergraduate needs.

This is the second edition, which is extensively revised, and even more focused on 'lists'. The relative importance and frequency of conditions are included. A feature of the book is an outline of the basic management of common and important acute clinical situations which may come up in the clinical examination or oral. These are necessarily brief and selected and no attempt has been made to surplant the conventional texts.

If these efforts of mine ease the pain of children *and* candidates, I shall be well rewarded!

Isleworth, 1995                                                    A.H.

# Contents

# Introduction

## GENERAL HINTS ON PHYSICAL EXAMINATION

1. **Observation**

   The toddler, especially if a 'terrible 2' year old, is unlikely to cooperate fully. Balance, gait, dexterity and speech can often be assessed by indirect observation while taking a history. The examiner may ask for your observations.

2. **Engaging the child**

   Start with the parent. The child is more likely to be approachable if a friendly rapport is established between you and an adult he knows and trusts. Opening gambits such as 'How are you?' and 'How old are you?' or questions about travel, school, favourite TV programmes, pitched at an appropriate level, break the ice. Be friendly, smile! Toddlers often avoid direct eye gaze, or get upset if you look directly at them, so go along with them until they get used to you.

3. **Touching**

   Not infrequently, small children resent or even fear a stranger touching them. Start with the hands. A game like 'round and round the garden', or for the feet 'this little pig went to market', works well.

4. **Examining**

   Be gentle, doing 'easy' bits to begin with. Ears and throat or a rectal examination come last. Be an opportunist: do not expect to be allowed to do things in order.

   Undressing can be upsetting, so ask the parent, if one is present, to undress the child. Removing a single garment at a time usually maintains cooperation.

   Palpating the abdomen or listening to heart sounds by coming round from behind the child, out of sight, may be successful in the fretting infant.

Demonstration of auscultation or looking at the ear on an adult, especially a parent, helps. Let the child play with your torch, sphygmomanometer bulb, stethoscope, etc. A toy given to the infant before attempting auscultation will distract him from pulling the stethoscope away during the procedure.

5. **Height, weight and head circumference measurements**
   Always obtain these measurements and plot them on a centile chart.

# Congenital abnormalities

**CAUSES OF CONGENITAL ABNORMALITIES**

*Common*
1. Unknown
2. Genetic
3. Chromosomal
*Uncommon*
4. Maternal
    (i) Drugs: thalidomide, norethisterone, antimetabolites
    (ii) Infection: cytomegalovirus, rubella, toxoplasmosis
    (iii) Metabolic: diabetes mellitus, phenylketonuria
    (iv) Exposure: radiation
5. Uterine
    (i) Moulding, e.g. talipes, dislocation of hips (CDH)
    (ii) Amniotic bands, e.g. amputations, facial clefts
    (iii) Early chorionic villous biopsy: moulding (i)

**INCIDENCE OF CONGENITAL MALFORMATIONS**

Major malformations: 1 in 50 of all live births.
Minor malformations: 1 in 25 of all live births.
    Association of two or more major malformations occurs in 1 in 10; therefore look carefully for abnormalities in other systems if one organ/system is affected.

## FETAL DEVELOPMENT AND MALFORMING (TERATOGENIC) AGENTS

### Teratogenic agents related to stage of fetal development

| Age and stage of development | Teratogens and their effects |
| --- | --- |
| 0–3 weeks old, early embryo | Chromosomal abnormality or abortion likely from irradiation and antimetabolites |
| 4–9 weeks old, stage of organogenesis | Abortion<br>Major malformation, e.g:<br>   Thalidomide: phocomelia<br>   Alcohol: fetal alcohol syndrome<br>   Infection (toxoplasmosis, cytomegalovirus (CMV) and rubella): mental handicap, microcephaly, small for dates, deafness, cataracts (not in toxoplasmosis), and (in rubella) heart defects |
| 10–40 weeks fetal growth | Altered growth and organ injury, growth failure, e.g.:<br>   Stilboestrol: vaginal carcinoma<br>   CMV: encephalitis, pneumonia, hepatosplenomegaly |

## MODES OF INHERITANCE

### Autosomal dominant
Recurrence risk 1 in 2 if:
1. One parent has the disease, e.g. adult polycystic kidney, spherocytosis, Huntingdon's chorea
2. Neither parent affected, i.e. spontaneous mutation, is common, and the risk to the affected child's offspring is 1 in 2, e.g. achondroplastic child with normal parents
3. Grandparent and grandchild affected, 'skipped generation', i.e. parent appears normal or is slightly affected, e.g. von Recklinghausen's disease, or detected only by special investigation, e.g. a computed tomogram of the brain showing characteristic calcification in tuberous sclerosis

### Autosomal recessive
Recurrence risk 1 in 4.
   Each parent carries a single abnormal gene for a disease found only when present in a double dose. This is thus more likely in consanguineous unions.
   Examples: sickle cell disease, thalassaemia, cystic fibrosis, inborn errors of metabolism.

## Sex linked
Usually recessive, risk to boys 1 in 2. A condition carried on the X chromosome, which males show as they have only one in each cell. Female carriers appear relatively or completely normal unless only one X is present, as in Turner's syndrome (XO). Lyon's hypothesis is that only one X chromosome is 'active' in each cell, and the number of active abnormal Xs a carrier has determines whether she shows any signs of the disease.
Mother carrier:  1 in 2 boys affected
1 in 2 girls carriers
Father affected: All boys normal
All girls carriers
   Examples: colour blindness (8% of boys), glucose-6-phosphate dehydrogenase deficiency, X-linked mental retardation (commonest cause of retardation in boys), haemophilia, Duchenne's muscular dystrophy.

## Multifactorial inheritance
Interaction of an individual's genes with the environment. The likelihood of recurrence (risk) increases as the number of family members affected increases, at a rate peculiar to that condition.
   Example: spina bifida (vitamin/folic acid lack in genetically susceptible individuals), recurrence risk for parents:
   Risk for the general population = <1 per 1000
   Risk of another after 1 affected child born = 1 in 20
   Risk after 2 affected children born to them = 1 in 8

## 'High' and 'low' risk in genetic counselling
For the purpose of counselling, geneticists suggest that a recurrence rate of more than 1 in 10 is a high risk, e.g. autosomal dominant, recessive and X-linked disease. A low risk is <1 in 10, e.g. insulin-dependent diabetes (about 1 in 10 to 1 in 20 in brothers, sisters and offspring of affected person).
   The example of multifactorial inheritance, spina bifida, shows how a family's category of risk can change.

## Gene probes
To identify individuals, affected or carriers. These probes may be single for a point gene mutation such as sickle cell anaemia, thalassaemia, haemophilia, or multiple where the gene locus is not yet identified but sites close to it are, e.g. Huntingdon's chorea.

## Gene mutations

Over 250 mutations have been identified for cystic fibrosis (CF). The gene for CF lies on chromosome 7. In 70% of CF cases in the UK, a single triplet codon for phenylalanine (F) is missing at position 508 on the protein called cystic fibrosis transmembrane conductance regulator (CFTR). CFTR is not as good as normal at allowing sodium and chloride ions to pass across the cell membranes. The defect is written as $\triangle$F 508 CFTR. Disease manifestations and severity are related to genotype.

## Incidence of some commoner congenital abnormalities

| | |
|---|---|
| Cleft lip and palate | 1 in 1000 births |
| Talipes eqinovarus | 1 in 1000 births |
| Congenital dislocation of the hips: | F = 1 in 1000 births |
| | M = 1 in 10 000 births |
| Pyloric stenosis | M = 1 in 200 infants |
| | F = 1 in 600 infants |

## Interventions to reduce incidence of anomalies

| Condition | Intervention |
|---|---|
| Spina bifida | Folic acid orally near conception |
| | Alpha fetoprotein (AFP) estimation |
| | Fetal ultrasound scan |
| Down's syndrome | Fetal ultrasound for 'nuchal oedema' |
| | Triple test (AFP, oestriol, human |
| | gonadotrophin hormone) |

## SOME SELECTED CHROMOSOMAL ABNORMALITIES

### 1. Down's syndrome

Frequency: 1 in 600 live births, 1 in 50 in 40-year-old mothers. Non-disjunction at meiosis is commonest with 47 chromosomes, and is sporadic in 95% of cases with 1% recurrence risk. Translocation of whole/part of one chromosome onto another is uncommon: karyotype is 46 chromosomes, found in 3% of cases and likely to recur in 10–100% of offspring because one parent carries the abnormal chromosome and has a 45 chromosome karyotype.

Clinical: characteristic face, hands and feet. Hypotonia, mental retardation, congenital heart disease, duodenal atresia and Hirschsprung's disease.

**2. Turner's syndrome (XO)**
Frequency: 1 in 4000 live births, owing to loss of X or Y
chromosome and unlikely to recur.
Neonate: low birth weight, low hair line, redundant skin folds,
oedema of feet, coarctation of the aorta.
Childhood: *short stature*, cubitus valgus, webbed neck,
occasional learning disability. Ovarian dysgenesis causes failure of
pubertal development.

**3. Klinefelter's syndrome (XXY)**
Frequency: 1 in 2000 live births, recurrence unlikely.
Clinical: 'maleness' predominates because of the Y
chromosome. Normal looking as boys, may be mentally slow, often
tall. At puberty 'eunuch' like, with gynaecomastia, small infertile
testes, rounded hips.

**4. Familial fragile X syndrome in XY males (X-linked mental
retardation)**
Frequency: 1 in 1000 males, X-linked recessive, recurrence risk 1 in
2 for boys, carrier females may be mentally slow.
Clinical: speech delay, autistic traits educationally subnormal,
large ears and head, large testes in adults.

**5. XYY syndrome**
Frequency: 1 in 1000 males, recurrence unlikely.
Clinical: tall, otherwise normal looking. Behaviour often
aggressive, occasionally 'psychopathic.'

# Newborn

## DEFINITIONS AND MORTALITY RATE FOR 1992 IN ENGLAND AND WALES

*Stillbirth:* No sign of life immediately after expulsion from mother after the 24th week of gestation. Rate: 4.3 in 1000 total live and stillbirths after 28 weeks.

*Perinatal mortality:* Number of stillbirths and deaths in the first week. Rate: 7.5 in 1000 total live and stillbirths.

*Neonatal mortality:* Number of deaths in the first 28 days of life. Rate: 4.3 in 1000 live births.

*Postneonatal mortality rate:* Number of deaths from 1 month to the end of the first year. Rate: 2.2 in 1000 live births.

*Infant mortality:* Number of deaths in the first year. Rate: 6.5 in 1000 live births.

*Premature:* <37 weeks' completed gestation.

*Small for dates (SFD):* Below 10th centile for length, weight and/or head circumference.

*Postmature:* 42 or more weeks' completed gestation.

## MAJOR CAUSES OF NEONATAL MORTALITY

1. Respiratory distress syndrome
2. Immaturity    } Prematurity (65%)
3. Asphyxia, birth injury
4. Congenital abnormalities
5. Infection

## CAUSES OF POSTNEONATAL MORTALITY (deaths between 1 month and the end of the first year of life)

1. Sudden infant death syndrome
2. Congenital anomalies
3. Conditions originating in the perinatal period (e.g. bronchopulmonary dysplasia, hydrocephalus, infection)

## CAUSES OF ABNORMAL BEHAVIOUR (apathy, irritability, fits, etc.)

Neurological findings are influenced by alertness, satiety (hours before/after feed) and intercurrent illness.

*Common*
1. Hypoxia, birth injury
2. Drugs: therapeutic and addictive withdrawal
3. Infection: congenital and acquired
4. Intracranial haemorrhage: intraventricular, periventricular
5. Metabolic abnormality: acidosis, hypoglycaemia, inborn errors
*Less common*
6. Chromosome abnormality
7. Brain malformation
*Uncommon*
8. Neuromuscular disease, e.g. Prader-Willi syndrome

### Problems of the low-birthweight infant
Of the 7% of all babies born weighing <2.5 kg, 60% are premature and 40% are small for dates. Further categorization is by weight into:

    (i) very-low-birthweight baby (VLBW) below 1500 g. Mortality rates in 1991: perinatal 272, neonatal 212
   (ii) extremely-low-birthweight baby (ELBW) of <1000 g for the purpose of identifying and documenting the high risk, dependency and cost, and increased morbidity and mortality of these groups.

## PREMATURITY

### Definition
Born before 37 weeks' gestation.

### Causes
*Common*
1. Unknown (50%), linked to social disadvantage
2. Uterus
    (i) Abnormal, e.g. cervical incompetence
   (ii) Uterine distension, e.g. twins, polyhydramnios
  (iii) Premature rupture of membranes, includes (i)
3. Antepartum haemorrhage: abruption, placenta praevia
4. Maternal
    (i) Teenage: reduced antenatal care, increased toxaemia
   (ii) Previous premature delivery
  (iii) Closely spaced pregnancies
  (iv) Acute maternal illness, infection, drug addiction
5. Fetal: congenital malformation, infection
6. Elective delivery or iatrogenic: eclampsia and toxaemia, Rhesus isoimmunization, diabetes, fetal distress, accidentally after fetoscopy

**Problems of the premature**
*Early (common)*
1. Immaturity
    (i) Respiration
        (a) Central control unstable (apnoea)
        (b) Surfactant deficiency (respiratory distress syndrome)
        (c) Alveolar–arteriolar gradient in the ELBW due to columnar epithelium, and underdeveloped pulmonary vascular beds
    (ii) Cardiovascular: bradycardias, hypotension, cardiac failure due to patent ductus arteriosus from early fluid excess (in the first 3 days) or reopening with hypoxia or anaemia
    (iii) Feeding: absent gag reflex before 34 weeks, functional ileus
    (iv) Liver: jaundice
2. Hypothermia: lack of brown fat and subcutaneous fat layer
3. Hypoglycaemia: lack of liver glycogen stores
4. Intraventricular haemorrhage: the less mature the more likely. Linked to metabolic acidosis, hypoxia, fluctuations in blood pressure
5. Infection
6. Necrotizing enterocolitis
7. Iatrogenic
8. Hyponatraemia: relative inability of the VLBW kidneys to conserve sodium

*Later (common unless anticipated and early treatment instituted)*
1. Anaemia
    (i) Early dilutional = normochromic at 4–6 weeks
    (ii) Late nutritional = hypochromic at 8–12 weeks
    (iii) Haemolytic = folic acid deficiency, vitamin E deficiency
2. Metabolic bone disease of prematurity
    (i) Probably inadequate phosphorous and/or calcium intake in VLBW infants
    (ii) Classical rickets: lack of vitamin D more likely from premature infants' rapid growth rate
3. Persistent patent ductus arteriosus: early fluid overload
4. Oxygen toxicity: retrolental fibroplasia and bronchopulmonary dysplasia in which trauma from mechanical ventilation also implicated
5. Brain damage: cerebral palsy, hydrocephalus from intra-ventricular haemorrhage. Less overt in VLBW: Learning disability, hearing loss
6. Growth potential: may be diminished in the VLBW
7. Bonding failure with parents

## SMALL FOR DATES (SFD)

### Definition
Below the 10th centile for weight. These infants may be symmetrically small in all body proportions or light for dates (LFD), i.e. length and head circumference above the 10th centile.

### Causes
1. Symmetrically small: early interference with fetal growth before 25 weeks' gestation
    (i) Fetal
        (a) Chromosomal abnormalities, e.g. trisomy 21, XO
        (b) Congenital abnormality
        (c) Fetal infection: cytomegalovirus, toxoplasmosis, rubella
    (ii) Maternal
        Drugs, e.g. chronic alcoholism, heroin addiction
2. Small in height and/or weight, usually with sparing of head growth. Attributable to onset of chronic intrauterine malnutrition after 24 weeks' gestation
    (i) Maternal
        (a) Malnutrition, race, social disadvantage, etc.
        (b) Hypoxaemia, e.g. smoking, high altitude
    (ii) Placental insufficiency, e.g. renal, essential hypertension, sickle cell, toxaemia and placental infarction
    (iii) Inadequate space, e.g. multiple pregnancy

### Problems of the SFD infant
*Common*
1. Hypoxia
    (i) Intrauterine death during pregnancy or labour
    (ii) Polycythaemia
    (iii) Meconium aspiration causing pneumonia
2. Hypoglycaemia: inadequate glycogen stores, jittery, increased hunger drive
3. Hypothermia: lack of subcutaneous fat
4. Polycythaemia: results in jaundice, thromboses in the brain, heart failure, rarely pulmonary haemorrhage
5. Congenital/chromosomal/infection problems, i.e. examine very carefully!
6. Abnormal neurology: seizures (hypoglycaemia, hypoxia, hypocalcaemia), jitteriness, apathy

### Problems of the LFD infant
*Common*
1. Intrauterine: chronic hypoxia, intrauterine death
2. Intrapartum
    (i) Acute or chronic hypoxia → death
    (ii) Meconium aspiration

3. Postpartum
    (i) Behavioural jitteriness, excessive/diminished feeding ability
    (ii) Hypoglycaemia in first 12 hours
    (iii) Temperature instability, increased calorie requirements
    (iv) Polycythaemia: jaundice (rarely thromboses, cardiac failure)
*Rare*
4. Pulmonary haemorrhage

## BIRTH TRAUMA

1. Swellings and the usual time of identification
    (i) Caput: at birth
    (ii) Cephalohaematoma: 2–4 days old
    (iii) Fractured clavicle: 1–20+ days
    (iv) Sternomastoid tumour: 7–20+ days
    (v) Fat necrosis: 3–14 days
2. Common nerve palsies, usually identified at birth
    (i) Facial nerve, peripheral: asymmetrical crying face, open eye
    (ii) Erb's palsy C5,6, waiter's tip posture

## CONDITIONS ASSOCIATED WITH THE ONSET OF RESPIRATORY DISTRESS SYNDROME (RDS)

*Common*
1. Prematurity
2. Asphyxia, intrapartum aspiration, second twin
3. Maternal factors
    (i) Antepartum or intrapartum haemorrhage
    (ii) Caesarean delivery without labour
    (iii) Diabetes mellitus
4. Previous sibling with RDS

## CAUSES OF FAILURE TO ESTABLISH RESPIRATION

1. Neurological
*Common*
    (i) Maternal medication/sedation
    (ii) Asphyxia/birth injury
    (iii) Prematurity
2. Respiratory
*Common*
    (i) Laryngeal spasm due to vigorous pharyngeal suction
*Uncommon*
    (ii) Pneumothorax
    (iii) Massive meconium aspiration

*Rare*
    (iv) Small lungs, e.g. Potter's syndrome of absent kidney
        function, oligohydramnios, pulmonary hypoplasia and
        'squashed baby'
    (v) Diaphragmatic hernia
3. Metabolic
*Common*
    (i) Hypoglycaemia
    (ii) Acidosis
4. Circulatory = shock from blood loss
*Less common*
    (i) Internal: ruptured organ, into muscles, into subaponeurotic
        space
    (ii) Maternal
    (iii) Twin to twin

**Hyperoxia test**
Abolition of cyanosis, present while breathing room air, by
breathing 100% oxygen, makes parenchymal lung disease likely
and congenital heart disease or large vascular shunts unlikely.

**CAUSES OF RESPIRATORY DISTRESS, APNOEA AND CYANOSIS**

1. Respiratory
*Common*
    (i) Parenchymal: RDS, meconium aspiration, pneumonia,
        pneumothorax
*Uncommon*
    (ii) Congenital structural, upper airway: hypoplastic jaw + cleft
        palate (Pierre–Robin syndrome), choanal atresia,
        oesophageal atresia
    (iii) Congenital structural, lower airway: lung hypoplasia, lobar
        emphysema, diaphragmatic hernia
2. Cardiac
    (i) Cardiac failure
    (ii) Congenital heart disease
    (iii) Persistent fetal circulation: full term, moderately
        asphyxiated baby, normal heart and lungs, raised
        pulmonary vascular resistance
3. Neurological
    (i) Asphyxia/birth injury; CVA (intraventricular haemorrhage);
        drugs
    (ii) Epilepsy, i.e. seizures
4. Metabolic: hypoglycaemia, acidosis
5. Polycythaemia, anaemia (acyanotic)

## CAUSES OF APATHY, APNOEA, IRRITABILITY, SEIZURE

Aid to memory:
  **A**sphyxia
  **B**irth injury
  **C**ongenital/chromosomal
  **D**rugs and drug withdrawal
  **E**pilepsy (familial neonatal fits — rare)
  **F**ifth day fits (diagnosed by exclusion)
  **G**lucose and other metabolic causes, e.g. sodium, calcium, magnesium, acidosis, kernicterus, inborn errors
  **H**aemorrhage: intraventricular haemorrhage: premature, vitamin K deficiency, thrombocytopenia
  **I**mmaturity (prematurity)
  **I**nfection

## JAUNDICE

Clinically recognized at 100 μmol/l serum bilirubin. 'Direct' or conjugated bilirubin should be <25 μmol/l.

### Causes
* = conditions in which 'direct' bilirubin is raised.

1. First day
*Uncommon*
    (i) Rhesus isoimmunization, occasionally ABO incompatibility
    (ii) Infection*, congenital (TORCH) and acquired
2. First week
*Common*
    (i) Physiological
    (ii) Haemolytic
        (a) Blood group incompatibility: ABO, Rhesus, minor blood groups
        (b) Red cell abnormality, e.g. hereditary spherocytosis
        (c) Enzyme deficiency: glucose-6-phosphate dehydrogenase deficiency common in Asians, Africans and Chinese
    (iii) Polycythaemia: small for dates, late clamping of cord, feto-maternal and feto–fetal transfusion
    (iv) Extravisated blood reabsorption from bruises, cephalhaematoma, swallowed maternal blood
    (v) Infection*, congenital and acquired
    (vi) Gut obstruction: ileus, Hirschsprung's disease
    (vii) Metabolic: minor contributory causes, e.g. oxytocics, hypoglycaemia, dehydration

3. Late onset after 1 week
*Less common*
    (i) Breast milk jaundice
    (ii) Infection*: urinary tract infection, herpes, hepatitis
    (iii) Metabolic: hypothyroidism (1 in 7000)
*Rare but important*
    (iv) Biliary atresia*/neonatal hepatitis syndrome* (1 in 10 000)

## ANAEMIA

At birth a healthy mature infant's venous haemoglobin (Hb) is 19 g/dl; a premature infant's Hb is 16 g/dl. Anaemia: <14 g/dl in the first week.

**Causes**
*Common*
1. Haemorrhage
    (i) Into mother/twin
    (ii) Into baby: trauma, vitamin K deficiency
    (iii) Revealed: cord and placenta accidents, circumcision
2. Haemolysis
    (i) Infection, profound acidosis
    (ii) Rhesus (direct Coombs' test positive), ABO
    (iii) Red cell defects: G-6-PD, spherocytosis
    (iv) Haemoglobinopathies: Hb Barts, etc.
3. Iatrogenic (blood taking)
*Rare*
4. Inadequate production, due to hypoplastic RBC anaemia (Blackfan-Diamond)

## CAUSES OF BLEEDING

1. Sick infant
*Common*
    (i) Consumption coagulopathy: cold, hypoxia, acidosis, sepsis
    (ii) Vascular injury: ventricular bleed
    (ii) Mechanical platelet injury, e.g. necrotizing enterocolitis
2. Well infant
*Uncommon*
    (i) Maternal thrombocytopenia or platelet antibody
        isoimmunization
    (ii) Haemorrhagic disease (vitamin K deficiency): breast fed, maternal anticonvulsants

## CAUSES OF HYPOGLYCAEMIA

Normal values: generally taken as >2.2 mmol/l (40 mg/dl), regardless of gestation.

*Common*
1. Delayed or inadequate feeds
2. Inadequate stores
     (i) Prematurity
     (ii) Small for dates
3. Increased requirement
     (i) Stress: infection, RDS, hypothermia
     (ii) Hyperinsulinism: infant of diabetic mother

## CAUSES OF HYPOCALCAEMIA

<1.8 mmol/l.

1. Early, 0–3 days: low calcium, normal phosphate
*Common*
     (i) Prematures
     (ii) Asphyxia
     (iii) Small for dates
     (iv) Stress, e.g. RDS, sepsis, surgical
     (v) Infant of diabetic mother
2. Late, 4–21 days: low calcium and/or magnesium, elevated phosphate
     (i) Cow's milk (Asians especially vulnerable to relative maternal hyperparathyroidism due to dietary lack of vitamin D and calcium → fetal hypoparathyroidism)
*Rare*
     (ii) Maternal hyperparathyroidism, vitamin D deficiency, renal disease

## CAUSES OF VOMITING

1. First 1–3 days
*Very common/common*
     (i) Feeding problem
     (ii) Gastric irritation, swallowed blood
     (iii) Infection
     (iv) Neurological: asphyxia/birth injury, intraventricular haemorrhage
*Uncommon*
     (v) Obstruction: duodenal atresia (double bubble on X-ray), stricture or web, bands, mid-gut rotation, meconium ileus, meconium plug, Hirschsprung's disease, anal atresia
2. End of first week
*Common*
     (i) Hiatus hernia
     (ii) Infection

*Less common*
    (iii) Necrotizing enterocolitis
    (iv) Obstructive: pyloric stenosis, volvulus, anal stenosis, Hirschsprung's disease
*Uncommon*
    (v) Metabolic: renal failure, inborn errors of metabolism, e.g. congenital adrenal hyperplasia

## CAUSES OF DELAY IN PASSING MECONIUM

1. First day
*Common*
    (i)   Physiological, 95% of newborns do, but 5% take up to 48 hours
    (ii)  Organic obstruction: anal stenosis or atresia, vesicorectal malformations
    (iii) Motility disorders: prematurity, opiates
*Uncommon but important*
    (iv) Hirschsprung's disease
    (v) Metabolic: hypothermia
    (vi) Meconium plug, cystic fibrosis
2. Delay in passing stool on subsequent days
    (i) Underfeeding, vomiting
    (ii) Breast feeding, simple constipation
    (iii) Hypothyroidism

## CAUSES OF HAEMATEMESIS

*Common*
1. Swallowed maternal blood
2. Gastritis
3. Oesophagitis
4. Peptic 'stress' ulceration, duplication, Meckel's diverticulum
5. Iatrogenic trauma, e.g. nasogastric tubes, airways
*Less common*
6. Coagulation defect: vitamin K deficiency, consumption of factors, low platelet count
7. Necrotizing enterocolitis

## CAUSES OF BLOOD IN THE STOOL

*Common*
1. Swallowed maternal blood (may be profuse)
2. Infection (often with mucus)
3. No cause found
4. Trauma, local, e.g. hard stool
*Less common*
5. Cow's milk allergy (may be colitis-like)
6. Necrotizing enterocolitis (often profuse)
7. Haemorrhagic disease of the newborn (may be profuse)

## CAUSES OF ABDOMINAL SWELLING

*Common*
1. Renal: hydronephrosis or multicystic kidney in 80%
   (uncommon: posterior urethral valves, polycystic kidney)
*Uncommon*
2. Hepatosplenomegaly: heart failure, infections, bleed into the organ
3. Intestinal obstruction: meconium ileus, volvulus, intussusception, Hirschprung's disease

## CAUSES OF CARDIAC FAILURE
See page 52.

### Guthrie test
Routinely performed between 6th and 14th day of life.
Screens for:
1. Phenylketonuria
2. TSH level
Selected areas of the United Kingdom also screen for haemoglobinopathies.

## CAUSES OF IATROGENIC DISEASE

### Historical
1. Delayed feeding of prematures: early hypoglycaemia, later increased incidence of cerebral palsy, smaller head circumference
2. Deliberate hypothermia, incorrectly thought to reduce oxygen requirements. Increased mortality
3. Jaundice
   (i) Water soluble vitamin K causing haemolysis
   (ii) Drugs displacing bilirubin from albumin causing kernicterus, e.g. sulphonamides
   (iii) Drug inhibition of glucuronidation by novobiocin

### Still topical
1. Retinopathy of prematurity: oxygen toxicity plays a part
2. Chloramphenicol excess: 'grey baby syndrome' = shock due to cardiovascular collapse, seizures
3. Excessive separation of parents and infant
4. Vitamin K intramuscular injection and childhood leukaemia: not proven?

# Development and neurology

## NORMAL DEVELOPMENT

### SOME MILESTONES IN NORMAL DEVELOPMENT
Know at least one item per category for each age band

| Social | Hearing and speech | Vision and fine motor | Gross motor |
|---|---|---|---|
| **6 weeks**<br>1. Smiles (H)<br>2. Coos (H) | 1. Stills to mother's voice or toy bell | 1. Follows face in 90° arc<br>2. Stares intently | 1. Sat up: lifts head few seconds<br>2. Examiner's hand lifting from under the body: head in line with trunk<br>3. Primitive reflexes present (Moro, ATNR) |
| **6 to 9 months**<br>1. Objects go to mouth<br>2. Enjoys bath and 'bo!'(H)<br>3. No longer looks at hand; looks at foot<br>4. Chews on biscuit (H) | 1. 6 months: 'ma, da'<br>2. 9 months: babbles,<br>3. 'Mama, dada', understands 'no-no' , bye-bye'(H)<br>4. Responds to own name<br>5. Hearing test by distraction | 1. Eyes fix on pellet of paper<br>2. Falling object:<br>(i) at 6 months forgets to follow it with eyes<br>(ii) at 9 months follows it<br>3. 6 months: palmar grasp; 7 months: transfers; 9 months: index finger probing approach | 6 months:<br>1. Rolls from back to front<br>2. Sits alone few seconds<br>3. Flexes head and trunk when pulled to sit<br>9 months:<br>1. Sits securely<br>2. Pulls up on furniture to stand |

| Social | Hearing and speech | Vision and fine motor | Gross motor |
|---|---|---|---|
| **1 year** | | | |
| 1. Comes when called | 1. Shakes head for 'no' | 1. Picks up crumbs with pincer grasp | 1. Pivots when sitting |
| 2. Lets go on request; finds hidden item | 2. Understands some words; says 1 to 3 words (H) | 2. Throws toys deliberately, watching them fall to the ground | 2. Walks alone or one hand held |
| 3. Dress: cooperates, pushing arm through sleeve | | 3. Holds 1 inch cube in each hand, bangs together, may make 2 cube high tower | |
| **18 months** | | | |
| 1. Cup: lifts, drinks and puts down (H) | 1. Jargons++ | 1. Fisted grasp of pencil, scribbles | 1. Walks well |
| 2. Spoon: feeds self (H) | 2. Points to 3 parts of body | 2. Points at wants | 2. Throws toy without falling |
| 3. Bowel training started, urine soaked nappy discarded | 3. Obeys single command 'get your cup', etc | 3. Picks up threads, pins, etc, neatly | 3. Climbs stairs (H) |
| 4. Copies: dusting, washing up, sweeping (H) | 4. Says 6 words; Echolalia | 4. Turns pages in picture book, 2 at a time | |
| | | 5. Tower of 3–4 × 1 inch cubes | |
| **2 to 2¹/₂ years** | | | |
| 1. Toilet: dry reliably by day, and tells in time (H) | 1. Many words | 1. Drawing: imitates vertical and horizontal line and circle | 1. Runs |
| 2. No sharing, plays alone, tantrums (H), demanding (H) | 2. Phrase of 2–3 words (H) | 2. Tower: 6–8 cubes | 2. Kicks ball |
| 3. Imaginative play | 3. Knows name | 3. Book: turns one page at a time | 3. Jumps on the spot |
| | 4. Understands 'give dolly a drink', i.e has inner language | | 4. Stairs: 2 feet per tread |
| | | | 5. Trike: pushes with feet |

| Social | Hearing and speech | Vision and fine motor | Gross motor |
|---|---|---|---|
| **3 to 3¹/₂ years** | | | |
| 1. Toilet: pulls pants down and up alone (H) | 1. Gives full name, sex | 1. Colour matches 2+ colours correctly | 1. Stands on one leg momentarily |
| 2. Eating: fork and spoon together (H) | 2. Counts by rote to 10 | 2. Mature pencil grip; copies circle | 2. Stairs; adult style of ascent (H) |
| 3. Plays with other child, shares toy (H) | 3. Uses 'me', 'I', 'you' | 3. Identifies square, triangle, although cannot draw them | 3. Trike: can pedal (H) |
| | 4. Understands on, under, back of, etc | | |
| **4 to 5 years** | | | |
| 1. Toilet: wipes own bottom (H) | 1. Gives name, address, age | 1. Colours: matches 4+ | 1. Hops |
| 2. Eating: knife and fork (H) | 2. Counts to 10 | 2. Drawing: *4 years* copies cross and square, by *5 years* a triangle, draws a man with head, arms, legs and fingers | 2. Climbs trees (H) |
| 3. Dress: on and off unsupervised, except tie, laces(H) | 3. Grammar OK | | 3. Ball games, catch', etc (H) |
| 4. Plays by the rules, is competitive | 4. Articulation almost mature | | |

H = by history, objective enough for most cases; otherwise by direct observation

## VISION

### Acuity

| At birth | 1/30th adult | = 6/180 m (20/600 ft) |
|---|---|---|
| 1 month | 1/15th adult | = 6/90 |
| 6 months | 1/5th adult | = 6/30 |
| 3–5 years | Equivalent to adult | = 6/6 (20/20 ft) |

### Colour blindness
Affects 6% of boys.

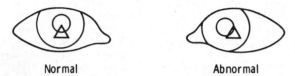

$\triangle$ = reflection of light source

Normal          Abnormal

**Fig. 1**

**Timing and nature of vision testing**
*Corneal light reflex*: Reflection of ophthalmoscope light is in the same spot on each eye. Overcomes the common confusion caused by epicanthus and wide nasal bridge. Fig. 1 shows abnormal reflection due to manifest squint.

NB: Resentment to covering one eye (the good one) may indicate abnormality in the other.

**Newborn.** Direct observation of eyes for abnormality; testing for the red reflex using an ophthalmoscope. Use +3 dioptres lens.
**6 Weeks.** History and mother's comments. Look for persistent squints (abnormal at any age), abnormal eye movements, lack of visual fixation of the face (delayed maturation, blind, autistic).
**6 Months.** Refer any squint to eye specialist; check eyes with ophthalmoscope.
**4 Years.** (i) Letter or symbol matching test, e.g. Sheridan-Gardiner 5 or 7 letter test.
(ii) Stereoscopic vision test.
**8 Years.** Colour vision testing.

**Causes of a red eye**
*Common*
1. Infection
    (i) Conjunctivitis
        (a) Neonatal: *N. gonorrhoea*, chlamydia, *S. aureus* (and silver nitrate prophylaxis)
        (b) Later: bacterial — *N. meningitidis, Strep. pneumoniae, S. aureus,* influenzae, leptospirosis
        viral — measles, chickenpox, adenovirus
    (ii) Keratitis: Herpes simplex, rarely H. zoster
    (iii) Endophthalmitis: metastatic spread of infection, e.g. group B β-streptococcus septicaemia in newborn

2. Allergic conjunctivitis, vernal conjunctivitis
3. Haemorrhage: traumatic, spontaneous, pertussis
4. Foreign body

## Causes of a painful eye, by quality and site
*Common*
1. Superficial foreign body sensation: corneal or conjunctival
    (i) Trauma, foreign body, contact lens
    (ii) Infection: conjunctivitis, keratitis
    (iii) Allergic and vernal conjunctivitis
    (iv) Exposure keratopathy, e.g. Bell's palsy, Down's syndrome
2. Burning or itching: conjunctival, allergy, lack of tears, chemical irritation
3. Orbital pain
    (i) Migraine, headache, sinusitis
    (ii) Rhabdomyosarcoma, retinoblastoma, abcess
*Rare*
4. Eyelid inflammation: stye, chalazion, cellulitis

## Causes of eyelid swelling
*Local causes (generally commonest)*
1. Inflammation: conjunctivitis, chalazion, stye, sinusitis (rarely cavernous sinus thrombosis)
2. Injury: direct trauma, foreign body, insect sting
3. Oedema: allergic, angioedema
(Uncommon local causes: capillary–cavernous haemangioma, neurofibroma)
*Systemic causes*
4. Systemic infection: roseola, scarlet fever, glandular fever, trichinosis
5. Generalized oedema: nephrotic syndrome, acute glomerulonephritis, cardiac failure

## Causes of amblyopia
*Definition*
Reduced visual acuity in one eye compared with the other, which if severe and uncorrected may result in permanent visual impairment.
1. Structural: corneal opacity, cataract, ptosis
2. Blurred image: refractive error, albinism
3. Squint

## Causes of squint
1. Non-paralytic (concomitant)
    (i) Failure of fusion of images (often inherited)
    (ii) Lens abnormalities (refractive errors, cataract)
    (iii) Nerve weakness due to febrile illness, head injury

2. Paralytic (incomitant)
   (i) Congenital: cranial nerve agenesis
   (ii) Tumour, false localizing sign in raised intracranial pressure

## Causes of blindness and partial sight
1. Cortical: damage to the occipital cortex and its connections due to trauma, meningitis, birth asphyxia, hydrocephalus
2. Eye: retinal degenerations, cataracts, optic atrophy, retrolental fibroplasia
3. Optic nerve or its radiation: tumour, trauma, cerebral palsy

## Causes of a white pupillary reflex
*Common*
1. Cataract
2. Congenital: coloboma, choroidoretinitis, etc.
*Uncommon*
3. Retinal detachment, e.g. non-accidental injury
4. Retrolental fibroplasia (retinopathy of prematurity)
5. Intra-ocular foreign body
6. Toxocara canis
7. Retinoblastoma

## HEARING

### Hearing tests
*Infancy*
Present quiet noises made with cup and spoon, rustling paper, high pitched rattle, whispered 's', 'oo' and baby's name. The head or eyes turn to the side tested
   7 months: at 50 cm from ear ⎫ 45 degrees behind baby's ear and
   9 months: at 1 m from ear    ⎭ level with it

*Preschool (2¹/₂ to 3 years old)*
1. Identifying objects: points to common objects, the names of which have already been said, then repeated at quieter sound levels during the test
2. 'Go' and 'sss' games: conditioning the child to place an object (toy) in a box each time you say 'go' or 'sss' at successively quieter sound levels

### Causes of deafness/failed hearing test
1. Acute otitis media  ⎫
2. Serous otitis media ⎭ conductive deafness
3. Congenital
   (i) Genetic, unknown — conductive and nerve deafness
   (ii) Infection, e.g. rubella, CMV — nerve deafness
4. Perinatal: asphyxia, hyperbilirubinaemia, drugs, prematurity — nerve deafness

## DEVELOPMENTAL WARNING SIGNS

1. Family history, e.g. deafness, cataracts
2. Mother worried
3. Motor problems
   (i) Persistence of reflexes (Moro, automatic walking, palmar grasp, tonic neck reflexes in cerebral palsy (CP) after time for disappearance)
   (ii) Early hand preference before 1 year, consider hemiplegia
   (iii) Not sitting unsupported by 9 months or walking by 18 months in CP, mental retardation, floppy baby (p 25)
   (iv) Boy not walking by 18 months: consider Duchenne's muscular dystrophy and test blood creatine phosphokinase activity (CPK)
4. Hearing and speech problems: see delayed speech (p 24)
   (i) No tuneful double syllable babble ('mumum, dadad') by 10 months
   (ii) <6 words at 18 months
   (iii) No 2–3 word sentences by 2 years
5. Visual difficulties (see p 20)
6. Social unresponsiveness: causes include deprivation, mental retardation, failure to thrive (p 33), autism

## CAUSES OF DELAYED DEVELOPMENT

By and large prematurity should be taken into account when assessing developmental progress, i.e. a 3 month premature infant at 6 months old will be at least a 3 month level of ability, usually more.
1. Idiopathic: constitutional, familial (affecting one field, e.g. bottom shuffler, catching up later)
2. Deprivation
3. Mental retardation
4. Specific abnormality, e.g. blind, deaf, cerebral palsy

## CAUSES OF DETERIORATION IN DEVELOPMENT

*Common*
1. Emotional shock, deprivation
2. Failure to thrive, intercurrent illness
3. Neurological: epilepsy, status epilepticus, drugs, any severe insult, e.g. trauma, meningitis
*Rare*
4. Metabolic: inborn errors, e.g. phenylketonuria, lead poisoning
5. Endocrine: hypothyroidism in infancy

## CAUSES OF PLAGIOCEPHALY (squint skull)

1. Intrauterine moulding
2. Lying mainly on one side: hypotonia, cerebral palsy
3. Sternomastoid shortening ('tumour')
4. Craniostenosis — premature fusion of one skull suture

## CAUSES OF A SMALL HEAD

1. Normal development: constitutional, familial, small body
2. Abnormal development likely: microcephaly
   (i) Familial and sporadic
   (ii) Brain injured: trauma, asphyxia, infection, etc.
   (iii) Mental retardation syndrome, e.g. Down's

## CAUSES OF A LARGE HEAD

1. Normal development: constitutional, familial (measure circumference of parents' heads)
2. Failure to thrive
3. Abnormal development likely
   (i) Hydrocephalus
   (ii) Subdural collections
   (iii) Tumour

## CAUSES OF DELAYED CLOSURE OF THE ANTERIOR FONTANELLE

(Normally achieved by 18–24 months)
1. Rickets
2. Hypothyroidism
3. Hydrocephalus

## CAUSES OF LEARNING DISABILITY (MENTAL HANDICAP)

1. Prenatal
   (i) Genetic:
      (a) Chromosomal, e.g. Down's syndrome, X-linked mental retardation (p 5)
      (b) Familial, e.g. tuberous sclerosis, inborn errors of metabolism
   (ii) Congenital infection: TORCH (p 2)
   (iii) Alcohol, drugs, e.g. phenytoin
2. Perinatal: asphyxia, birth injury, prematurity
3. Postnatal: meningitis, head injury, seizures, lead

## CAUSES OF SLOW SPEECH DEVELOPMENT

1. Deprivation, emotional
2. Developmental delay, often familial
3. Deaf, usually secretory otitis, others (p 22)

## CAUSES OF FLOPPY INFANTS

1. Non-neurological: failure to thrive, acute infection
2. Brain abnormality: injury, mental retardation, Down's syndrome, cerebral palsy
3. Spinal: trauma, polio, spinal muscular atrophy
4. Peripheral nerve: polyneuritis
5. Neuromuscular junction: myasthenia gravis
6. Muscular dystrophies

## CAUSES OF ABNORMAL GAIT PATTERN

*Common*
1. Limp (p 84): hemiplegia, joint disease
2. Broad-based gait: ataxia, dyskinetic cerebral palsy (CP)
*Uncommon*
3. Tip-toe: CP with scissoring of legs, muscular dystrophy, polyneuritis
4. Waddling gait: congenital dislocated hip, Duchenne muscular dystrophy, polymyositis, old polio peripheral neuropathy
5. Pes cavus: Friedrich's ataxia, spinal cord lesions
*Rare*
6. Foot drop: sciatic nerve damage, peroneal muscular atrophy, heavy metal poisoning

## CAUSES OF SEIZURES BY AGE

### Stage of brain maturation related to seizure type

| | |
|---|---|
| Neonatal (age up to 4 weeks) | Asphyxia/birth injury, infection, hypoglycaemia, hypocalcaemia, intracranial haemorrhage, drug withdrawal |
| Infantile spasms (age 3–9 months) | Idiopathic in 1/4 cases, tuberous sclerosis, brain malformations/injury, congenital infection, encephalopathy |
| Febrile convulsion (age 1–5 years) | Fever, usually due to infection and never, by definition, of the central nervous system, though it may need to be excluded |
| Petit mal (age 3–15 years) | Idiopathic |
| Benign focal epilepsy of childhood (age 7–10 years) | Idiopathic |

| Photosensitive epilepsy (age 8–14 years) | Idiopathic, but may be found in other forms of epilepsy and especially brain damage |
|---|---|

**Seizures largely independent of age**

| Grand mal | Genetic in many |
|---|---|

| Temporal lobe epilepsy | Idiopathic, genetic, or symptomatic of some underlying cause |
|---|---|

## CAUSES OF BACTERIAL MENINGITIS BY AGE

1. 0–3 months
   (i) Gram negative: *Escherichia coli*, proteus, pseudomonas
   (ii) Gram positive: group B streptococcus
2. Older ages
   (i) *Haemophilus influenzae* (now less comon due to Hib vaccination)
   (ii) *Neisseria meningitidis*
   (iii) *Streptococcus pneumoniae*
   (iv) Mycobacteriam tuberculosis (rare but important)

## CAUSES OF HEADACHE

1. Tension, especially likely in school refusal (p 28)
2. Migraine
3. Raised intracranial pressure: tumour, abscess
4. Post-traumatic
5. Infection: meningitis
6. Sinusitis, dental caries
7. Hypertension (rare)
8. Intracranial bleed (rare)

# Behaviour

**CAUSES OF ENURESIS**

1. Physiological delay (with family history usual)
2. Psychological stress
3. Organic
   (i) Urinary tract infection
   (ii) Mental retardation
   (iii) Neurological, e.g. spina bifida, epilepsy
   (iv) Structural lesion, e.g. posterior urethral valves
   (v) Diabetes mellitus

**CAUSES OF FAECAL SOILING**

1. Untrained
2. Organic: anal fissure resulting in constipation and overflow incontinence, Hirschsprung's disease
3. Psychological
   (i) Retention — may lead to fissure
   (ii) Antisocial

**CAUSES OF RECURRENT ABDOMINAL PAIN/PERIODIC SYNDROME**

1. Psychological stress
   (i) Home: marital discord, separation experiences, family illness, poor parent–child relationship
   (ii) School: bullying, problems in discipline and learning
   (iii) Sexual abuse
2. Migraine tendency: personal and family history
3. Constipation or *abnormal* bowel action
4. Medical causes of acute abdominal pain (p 59)

## CAUSES OF SCHOOL REFUSAL

1. School refusal: separation anxiety, refuses to leave home
2. Truancy (leaves home and fails to arrive or absconds later): educational difficulties, psychosocial problems common
3. Educational difficulties, e.g. slow, chronic illness, poor vision, unsuspected hearing loss, emotional stress, dyslexia, etc., poor teaching, large class

# Growth and nutrition

## NORMAL GROWTH: SOME CLINICAL RULES OF THUMB

1. Infant weight gain: 30 g/day (1 oz) from the 10th day
   Birth weight × 2 by 5 months
   Birth weight × 3 by 1 year
2. Tooth eruption, onset to completion
   Primary dentition      6 months to 2 years
   Permanent dentition   6 years to 12 years
   Third molars           20 years +

## NUTRITIONAL REQUIREMENTS FOR MAINTENANCE AND GROWTH

### Water
Daily oral requirments as milk (to provide adequate calories and enough water to excrete renal solute load mainly of urea and sodium)
Premature   up to 200 ml/kg/day
Neonate     150 ml/kg/day

Daily requirements, oral or intravenous, as water, are:
<10 kg      100 ml/kg/day
10–20 kg    50 ml/kg/day
>20 kg      20 ml/kg/day

### Calories
1. Up to 1 year: 460 kJ (110 kcal)/kg/day
   Prematures up to 580 kJ (140 kcal)/day
2. Subsequent years: 4200 kJ (1000 kcal) + 420 kJ (100 kcal) for each year of life
3. Calculate according to *expected* weight for gestational age and each year of life. Remember that 150 ml of milk contains 460 kJ (110 kcal)
4. Weaning: first solids introduced from 3–6 months. Unmodified door stop cow's milk from 12 months (not before as may result in iron deficiency)

## Vitamins
Recommended daily intake in the first year:

Term
          A 1500 IU
          C 30 mg
          D 400 IU

Premature (very low birth weight)
          A, B, C as above
          D 800 IU
          E 15 mg
          Folic acid 50 μg  } for 2–6 months

## Fluoride
Optimal fluoride concentration is 1 part per million (ppm) in tap water. Most toothpastes now contain fluoride.

## COMPARISON OF HUMAN, COW, AND MODIFIED MILKS

| Contents per 100 ml | Human | Cow | Modified |
| --- | --- | --- | --- |
| Calorie (kcal) | 70 | 67 | 65 |
| Carbohydrate (g) | 7 | 4.5 | 7 |
| Fat (g) | 4.2 | 3.9 | 3.5 |
| Protein (g) | 1.4 | 3.4 | 1.8 |
| Sodium (mmol/l) | 6 | 20 | 10 |

## HAZARDS OF COW'S MILK FEEDING
*Common*
1. Psychological for mothers, e.g. less satisfying, disappointed if unable to breast feed
2. Allergy: eczema, asthma, urticaria, anaphylaxis
3. Obesity, as more saturated fats than in breast milk

*Uncommon*
4. Infection
    (i) Preparation
    (ii) Lack of anti-infective factors
5. Electrolyte disorders: hypocalcaemia, hypernatraemia, metabolic acidosis, raised blood urea
6. Cow's milk protein intolerance: 5% of cases of infantile colic
7. Anaemia: occult bleeding

### Additional hazards of formula milks
Preparation
1. Overconcentration: hypernatraemia (historical?), obesity
2. Overdilution: marasmus
3. Anaemia, as symptom of cow's milk protein allergy

## BENEFITS OF BREAST FEEDING

1. Nutritionally balanced
2. Anti-infective properties: macrophages, lactoferrin, secretory IgA, lysosyme, lactobacilli (may be especially valuable for premature infants in prevention of infection and necrotizing enterocolitis)
3. Psychological
4. Anti-allergic

NB: Remember the hazards: early vitamin K deficiency, underfeeding, maternal medication excreted in breast milk. Infections include maternal HIV (a contraindication to breast feeding in developed countries, but not in underdeveloped countries) and hepatitis B, untreated maternal TB.

## NUTRITIONAL DISORDERS

### Vitamin A
A rare deficiency except in the developing world, still a major cause of blindness in some countries.
  Clinical: Night blindness, photophobia, dry corneas (xerophthalmia), keratomalacia; slow development; horny skin, respiratory infections.

### Scurvy
Lack of vitamin C results in bleeding gums, purpura from capillary bleeds, pseudo paresis due to subperiosteal bleeds.
  Exceedingly rare in developed countries.
Prevention: see p 30.
Treatment: 0.5 g vitamin C a day.

### Rickets
1. Due to vitamin D deficiency. At risk: Asian infants and adolescents, from inadequate intake, lack of sun, phytates in the diet; premature infants; less commonly, those taking anticonvulsants, malabsorbing (coeliac, etc.)
2. Vitamin D resistant rickets, renal rickets (chronic renal failure, renal tubular acidosis) — all rare
3. Substrate deficiency. Very-low-birth weight premature infants may be phosphate deficient
  Clinical: Frontal bossing, anterior fontanelle slow to close, enlarged wrists, swelling of rib ends ('rickety rosary'), symmetrical bow legs, hypotonic muscles
  Cause: In nutritional rickets low vitamin D intake causes inadequate calcium absorption from the gut; parathormone rises to mobilize calcium from bone and causes renal excretion of phosphate

Serum biochemistry shows:
  (a)  Calcium normal, phosphate low
  (b)  Alkaline phosphatase raised (upper limit in premature infants up to 5 times adult maximum, children twice that of adults, and again rising much higher in puberty)
  (c)  Vitamin D low
Radiology shows:
  (a)  Loss of normal bone density
  (b)  'Cupped' appearance at end of long bones due to widening of metaphysis
  (c)  Irregular calcification of the epiphyseal plate
  (d)  Greenstick fractures
Prevention: see p 30.
Treatment: 1500 IU vitamin D a day.

## Anaemia
Iron lack in premature infants, twins, delayed weaning. Pale, increased respiratory rate, palpable spleen, systolic murmur.

## Marasmus
Lack of protein and *calories*
Causes:
1. Placental, in utero (see small for dates — p 9)
2. Postinfective diarrhoea
3. Chronic infection e.g. UTI, TB, malaria
4. Malabsorption (e.g. cystic fibrosis)
5. Neglect

Clinical: Hungry unhappy infant, no oedema; length and weight below 3rd centile, i.e. stunted due to prolonged starvation; more acute weight loss results in 'baggy' skin folds.

Treatment: Feed to *expected* weight for height, high calorie and protein formula, avoid hypothermia, investigate for associated infection/ deficiency of iron, vitamins and possible cause. In developing countries education may prevent this.

## Kwashiorkor
Lack of protein greater than calories, i.e. at weaning in developing countries, 1–3 years old. Black skin depigments irregularly, hair reddens, generalized oedema, large liver, prone to infection, which often precipitates kwashiorkor.

## Obesity
Causes
1. Overeating
2. Constitutional, familial and racial
3. Emotional, compensatory overeating
4. Endocrine, e.g. Cushing's syndrome — iatrogenic from steroids. Beware the short fat child!

# GROWTH

## Measurement

A single measurement of height and weight allows a static comparison with the rest of the population using a standard growth chart.

Repeated measurements allow assessment of the rate of growth or growth velocity. The minimum interval between such measurements is 6 months using a stadiometer.

*Parental height comparison* will show whether the child is on the expected mid-parental centile, which can be roughly calculated from the standard chart as follows:

Boys   (i) Plot mother's height on the right hand margin
      (ii) Add 12.5 cm to this, make a mark
     (iii) Plot father's height, make a mark
     (iv) Expected height centile is mid point between the two marks

Girls   (i) Plot father's height and deduct 12.5 cm, mark
     (ii) Expected height centile is mid-way between the mark and mother's height

*BONE AGE* is the expected 'average' skeletal maturity at a given chronological age, both expressed in 'years'. Use in assessing cause of abnormal growth pattern.

1. Normal bone age, i.e. same as chronological age in short stature of family or genetic cause
2. Delayed bone age proportional to actual height, i.e. the height plotted on the chart at that bone age is within expected centiles (Fig. 2)
3. Delayed bone age, the actual height progressively falling away from expected velocity in failure to thrive (see below), hypothyroidism, growth hormone deficiency (Fig. 3). Without treatment final adult height may be reduced
4. Advanced bone age in virilization and precocious puberty (p 36)

*CATCH-UP growth* occurs for a finite period after suppression by subnutrition or severe illness and is an increased growth velocity towards expected stature.

## CAUSES OF SHORT STATURE/FAILURE TO THRIVE

1. *Common causes*
   (i) Undernutrition
  (ii) Constitutional: individual and familial
 (iii) Psychosocial deprivation
 (iv) Small for dates from pregnancy-induced hypertension (toxaemia)

HEIGHT CHART USING BONE AGE

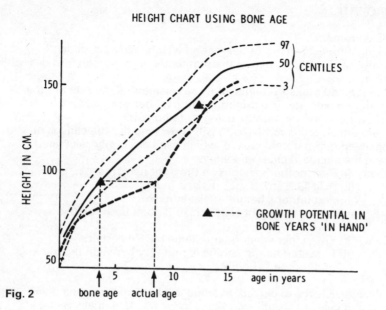

**Fig. 2**

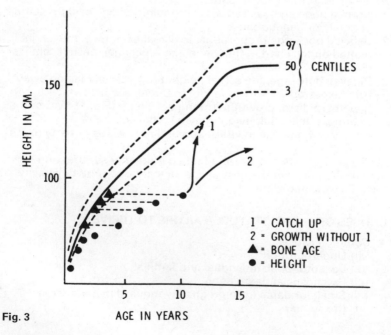

**Fig. 3**

(v) Malabsorption: intestinal infection, tropical infestation, coeliac, cystic fibrosis, Hirschsprung's disease
(vi) Mental retardation (microcephaly)
(vii) Iatrogenic: steroids (asthma/nephrotic/rheumatoid)
2. *Less common causes*
(i) Systemic disease: cyanotic congenital heart disease, cystic fibrosis, severe asthma, chronic renal failure
(ii) Chronic infection: malaria
(iii) Skeletal disorders: achondroplasia, rickets
3. *Rare causes*
(i) Endocrine: hypothyroidism, hypopituitarism, sexual precocity, Cushing's — including iatrogenic from steroids
(ii) Chromosomal: XO, Down's syndrome
(iii) Metabolic
(a) Genetic, e.g. glycogen storage
(b) Acquired, e.g. renal tubular acidosis

## CAUSES OF SHORT STATURE (after Charles Brook)

**Normal looking**
*Common*
1. Normal growth velocity
(i) Low birth weight
(ii) Short parents
(iii) Constitutional growth delay
2. Low growth velocity
(i) Psychosocial deprivation
(ii) Generalized disease, e.g. malabsorption, metabolic and systemic disease

**Distinguishing features**
*Uncommon*
1. Disproportionate growth
(i) Short trunk, e.g. spondylo-epiphyseal dysplasia
(ii) Short limbs, e.g. achondroplasia
2. Growth disorder syndromes, e.g. Turner's, Russell-Silver syndrome

## CAUSES OF TALL STATURE

1. Constitutional: individual, familial
2. Endocrine, e.g. precocious puberty (at first) (p 36), thyrotoxicosis,
congenital adrenal hyperplasia (p 39)
3. Chromosomal: XXY, XYY (p 5)
4. Marfan's syndrome

# Sexual differentiation and puberty

## SOME NORMAL PUBERTAL EVENTS

### Girls
1. Onset from 8–14 years with breast, genital, then pubic hair the usual order of development
2. Maximum growth achieved before menarche, only 6 cm on average after onset of menses
3. Menarche mean age is 13 years. The bone age at which menarche occurs corresponds to that at 13 years old

### Boys
1. The first sign of puberty is usually testicular enlargement at 10–14 years with an increase in volume to 4 ml (about a medium sized or stuffed olive). Accurate estimation is obtained with an orchidometer, a string of ovoids of increasing volume 1–24 ml, used for comparison by palpation
2. Gynaecomastia is common and normal and may be unilateral
3. The sex difference in height is largely due to 2 extra years' prepubertal growth because boys, on average, start puberty 2 years later

## PRECOCIOUS PUBERTY

Present if pubertal changes occur before 8 years in girls, 9 years in boys; commoner in girls. Pathological cause more likely in boys (60%) than girls (20%).

NB: Early breast development (premature thelarche) from 1–2 years old and axillary or pubic hair alone (adrenarche) from 7 years old is usually normal.

**Causes of precocious puberty**
1. True (mediated through gonadotrophins)
    (i) Physiological: constitutional, familial, obesity
    (ii) Hypothalamic: injury, hydrocephalus, postinfective, tumour
    (iii) Tumour producing gonadotrophins
2. False, or pseudo (sex hormones present in excess independent of hypothalamic or gonadotrophin control). Boys' testes remain small unless true precocious puberty due to tumour. Girls may be virilized.
    (i) Adrenal, e.g. congenital adrenal hyperplasia (p 39)
    (ii) Gonadal tumours of testes or ovaries
    (iii) Drug: anabolic steroids

## DELAYED PUBERTY

Absence of any signs by 14 years old, or prolonged arrest of progress after the initiation of puberty.

**Causes**
1. Physiological: constitutional or familial
2. Chronic disorders, e.g. malnutrition, coeliac, Crohn's disease, diabetes mellitus, anorexia nervosa
3. Hypothalamic/pituitary lack of gonadotrophins
4. Gonads unable to produce sex hormones despite adequate gonadotrophins, e.g. streak ovaries in Turner's syndrome
5. End organs unresponsive, e.g. testicular feminization

## VAGINAL DISCHARGE

Clear or white discharge in small amounts is physiological, and may cause a stain on the pants.

**Causes**
1. Physiological
2. Non-specific vaginitis
3. Infection: gonococcal, streptococcal, monilia, herpes, threadworm
4. Foreign body

## CAUSES OF AMBIGUOUS GENITALIA

1. Virilization of girls: congenital adrenal hyperplasia (p 39)
2. Feminization of boys
   (i) Undescended testes: normal, anorchia, XXY
   (ii) Testicular feminization: an X-linked disorder of end organ unresponsiveness to testosterone in an XY person — short blind ended vagina, no uterus, little pubic hair, testis may be found in inguinal hernia
   (iii) Errors in testosterone synthesis
3. Hermaphrodite, i.e. mixed gonads often with mosaic sex chromosomes

# Endocrinology

## AGE OF ONSET OF ENDOCRINE PROBLEMS

### Neonatal — infancy

1. Infant of diabetic mother
   Longer and heavier than expected, early hypoglycaemia, respiratory distress syndrome and jaundice more likely, higher incidence of congenital anomalies, e.g. sacral agenesis (absent sacrum)
2. Hypothyroidism
   Goitre — mother taking antithyroid drugs, familial disorders of thyroid synthesis; prolonged neonatal jaundice in a large baby likely
   Later in infancy: constipated, feeding difficulties, hypotonic, growling slow cry, pale (anaemia), coarse skin and hair, cold, large tongue, umbilical hernia, delayed bone age and general development slow, poor growth, thyroid stimulating hormone (TSH) level raised on Guthrie test, low thyroxine (T4)
3. Congenital adrenal hyperplasia (CAH)
   21-hydroxylase deficiency commonest, inherited in autosomal recessive mode, results in low cortisol, high androgen (male sex hormone) production, causing
   (i) Virilization of girls, and deeply pigmented genitals in boys at birth
   (ii) Shock from salt loss, with vomiting, dehydration, poor weight gain and lethargy from end of first week of life
   (iii) Sudden unexpected death
   Later: accelerated growth and pseudo-precocious puberty (p 37). Final adult height shorter if untreated.
   Biochemistry: raised serum potassium, urea; lowered sodium, bicarbonate; occasionally hypoglycaemia.
   Very high serum 17-hydroxyprogesterone best test for 21-hydroxylase deficiency in the neonate.

## Preschool (1–4 years)
Growth hormone deficiency, idiopathic
Commoner in boys, fall off in growth from beginning of second year, often insidious. Short, fat, large looking head, small genitals, well. May not be recognized until school age. Growth velocity <5 cm a year. Bone age not always delayed.

## School age
1. Diabetes mellitus, insulin dependent. Few days or weeks of poor appetite, weight loss, polydipsia, onset enuresis, monilial vulvitis, short history of vomiting, abdominal pain, deep sighing breathing, coma
   Investigation and treatment: see p 99
2. Hypothyroidism
   Causes: failing, small thyroid; autoimmune disease; lack of iodine (see goitre)
   Growth retarded with 'infantile' proportions (long trunk, short legs); bone age (p 33) retarded; excessively well behaved, no retardation in intellect; pale, constipated, dry skin, etc.; occasionally precocious puberty
3. Hyperthyroidism
   Diffusely enlarged thyroid; accelerated growth, advanced bone age; in addition to usual signs in adults, affecting the eyes and metabolism, early symptoms include disturbed behaviour, deterioration in handwriting and schooling
4. Cushing's syndrome
   Cause: commonly caused by iatrogenic steroid administration, e.g. for asthma, Still's disease
   Growth failure, osteoporosis; immunosuppression, increased danger from infection; adrenal suppression; moon face, buffalo hump, obese trunk, hirsute, acne; thin limbs from muscle wasting and weakness, personality change; hypertension; red face (high Hb), striae

## CAUSES OF GOITRE

1. Euthyroid
   (i) Physiological at puberty
   (ii) Autoimmune thyroiditis (later hypothyroid)
2. Hypothyroid
   (i) Iodine deficiency
   (ii) Antithyroid drugs
   (iii) Enzyme deficiency, usually familial
3. Hyperthyroid: thyrotoxicosis

## CAUSES OF HYPOGLYCAEMIA

Neonatal: p 14
Older ages: p 82

# Respiratory disease

## COMMON CAUSES OF RESPIRATORY DISEASE

Relationship of respiratory disease to age and common causes

| Disease | Age | Causal agents |
| --- | --- | --- |
| 1. Recurrent otitis media, upper respiratory tract infections | All ages | *Streptococcus pneumoniae, H. influenzae*, respiratory syncytial virus (RSV), adenovirus, influenza, parainfluenza |
| 2. Epiglottitis | 3–7 years | *H. influenzae* |
| 3. Laryngotracheo bronchitis | 1–3 years | RSV, parainfluenza, influenza, rhinoviruses |
| 4. Bronchiolitis | Infant | RSV |
| 5. Asthma | >1 year | Viruses; exercise/cold air, allergies; emotion, smoking |
| 6. Pneumonia | Neonate | *E. coli*, pseudomonas species, Group B haemolytic streptococcus |
| | Infant | RSV, influenza, *Staphylococcus aureus, Strep. pneumoniae* |
| | Child | RSV, influenza, parainfluenza, *Strep. pneumoniae, Mycoplasma pneumoniae* |

Relationship of age to infectious respiratory illness

| Age | Illness | Bacteria/protozoa | Viruses |
|---|---|---|---|
| Neonatal | Pneumonia | E. coli<br>Pseudomonas<br>Group B Haem. strep | Respiratory<br>syncitial<br>virus (RSV) |
| Infancy | Wheeze-related<br>viral infections | | RSV<br>Parainfluenza<br>Adenovirus<br>Rhinovirus |
| | Broncho-<br>pneumonia | Staph. aureus<br>Strep. pneumoniae<br>Pneumocystis<br>carinii (HIV) | Parainfluenza<br>Adenovirus<br>Rhinovirus<br>Influenza<br>Measles |
| Toddler<br>(1–3 years) | Laryngotracheitis<br>Broncho-<br>pneumonia | Strep. pneumoniae | As in infancy |
| | Asthma | Mycoplasma<br>pneumonia<br>(uncommon) | Rhinovirus<br>RSV<br>Parainfluenza,<br>etc. |
| 3–7 years | Epiglottitis | Haemophilus<br>influenzae | Parainfluenza<br>Influenza<br>Adenovirus<br>RSV |
| School age<br>(4+ years) | Broncho-<br>pneumonia | Strep. pneumoniae<br>Mycoplasma<br>pneumoniae<br>Measles | Adenovirus<br>Parainfluenza<br>Influenza |
| All ages | Recurrent<br>otitis media,<br>upper respiratory<br>tract infection | Strep. pneumoniae<br>H. influenzae | RSV<br>Adenovirus<br>Influenza<br>Parainfluenza |

## CAUSES OF ACUTE COUGH

Common
1. Acute upper and lower respiratory tract infection
2. Asthma
Uncommon
3. Foreign body
4. Pertussis

## CAUSES OF CHRONIC COUGH

*Common*
1. *Postnasal* drip: infected or atopic adenoids and sinuses
2. Asthma
3. Persistent infections: pertussis syndrome, *M. pneumoniae*, tuberculosis (TB), *Pneumocystis carinii* (HIV)
4. Habit
*Uncommon*
5. Foreign body
6. Aspiration syndromes: hiatus hernia
*Rare*
7. Cystic fibrosis, psittacosis

## CAUSES OF NOSE BLEEDS

*Common*
1. Trauma, nose picking
2. Infection
3. Allergic rhinitis
4. Foreign body
*Uncommon*
5. Bleeding disorders, vascular abnormality

## DIFFERENTIATION OF THE MAJOR CAUSES OF ACUTE STRIDOR

Epiglottitis (E), laryngotracheobronchitis (LTB) and foreign body (FB) above the carina

|  | E | LTB | FB |
|---|---|---|---|
| Age | 0–3 years | 3–7 years | >6 months |
| Onset | In hours | 1–2 days | Sudden, may be missed |
| Respirations | Laboured | Increased | Variable |
| Cough | + | + + | + + + |
| Drooling | + + + | — | — |
| Appearance | Pale, toxic | Normal/anxious | Normal |
| Voice | Hoarse, weak | Hoarse | May be aphonic |
| Hypoxia | Frequent | Unusual | Variable |
| X-ray of neck | Large epiglottis | Normal | Radio-opaque, FB? |
| Chest X-ray | Normal | Inflammatory changes in half the children | Lung or lobe overinflated/ collapsed if FB moves below carina |

## CAUSES OF ACUTE STRIDOR

1. Acute laryngotracheobronchitis
2. Acute epiglottitis
3. Foreign body
4. Rare but important: diphtheria, retropharyngeal abscess, acute angioneurotic oedema

**Foreign body: the level of obstruction of the respiratory tract and related timing of symptoms**

| Level of obstruction | Timing of onset | Symptoms |
| --- | --- | --- |
| **Laryngeal/tracheal** | | |
| (i) Mechanical obstruction | Immediate | Cough |
| (a) large, e.g. coin | | Stridor, aphonia, |
| (b) oedema: small, sharp | | dyspnoea, |
| object, e.g. a pin | | cyanosis |
| (ii) Chemical inflammation due to vegetable fibres | Hours to days | Wheeze or pneumonia |
| **Lower respiratory tract** e.g. roasted peanut, grass seed | Hours, days, weeks | Wheeze, unresolved infection or lung collapse, chronic cough |

## CAUSES OF CHRONIC STRIDOR

*Common*
1. Weak cartilage in the wall: laryngomalacia
2. Internal narrowing: subglottic stenosis after prolonged intubation in prematures
*Rare*
3. Compression from surrounding structures: vascular ring, tumour

## CAUSES OF RECURRENT WHEEZE

*Common*
1. Reactive airways: asthma/wheezy bronchitis/bronchiolitis
*Uncommon*
2. Mechanical:
    (i) Aspiration, e.g. hiatus hernia
    (ii) Foreign body, compression from mediastinal glands, masses
3. Cardiac failure
*Rare*
4. Genetic: cystic fibrosis

## CAUSES OF ACUTE RESPIRATORY FAILURE

| | Obstructive (common) | Restrictive (uncommon) | Diffusion defect (uncommon) | CNS depression (common) |
|---|---|---|---|---|
| **Upper** | Epiglottitis, stenosis, aspiration, laryngospasm | Pneumothorax Scoliosis Ascites (Rare: diaphragmatic hernia, small chest) | Interstitial pneumonitis (HIV) Pulmonary oedema | Drugs Trauma Encephalitis Asphyxia |
| **Lower** | Pneumonia, aspiration | | | |

## CAUSES TO CONSIDER CYSTIC FIBROSIS

1. Respiratory
    (i) Second pneumonia in infancy (or first if staphylococcal)
    (ii) Frequent bronchitis
    (iii) Pseudomonas chest infection
    (iv) *Staphylococcal pneumonia*
2. Growth and bowel problems
    (i) Meconium ileus
    (ii) Failure to thrive
    (iii) Rectal prolapse
3. Family history and asymptomatic

## CAUSES OF LYMPHADENOPATHY

*Common*
1. Normal to have small glands in the various sites
2. Infection
3. Eczema
*Uncommon/rare*
4. Malignancy
5. Drugs, serum sickness
6. Systemic juvenile chronic arthritis (Still's disease)

## X-RAY DIFFERENCES BETWEEN CONSOLIDATION AND COLLAPSE (ATELECTASIS)

|  | Consolidation | Collapse |
|---|---|---|
| Mediastinal shift | — | + Towards lesion |
| Compensatory hyperinflation of other lobes | — | + |
| Fissure position | Unchanged | + Towards lesion |
| Diaphragm on same side | Unchanged | Elevated |
| Air bronchogram | + | Variable |

## Causes of opaque hemithorax on X-ray

*Common*
1. Pneumonia
2. Aspiration
3. Complete collapse of a lung
4. Pleural effusion, empyema

# Cardiology

## NORMAL VALUES

| Age (years) | Heart rate (beats per minute) | Blood pressure (mm Hg) |
|---|---|---|
| 0–2 | 100–120 | 80/50–90/60 |
| 3–5 | 100 | 90/60 |
| > 5 | 80–90 | 90/60–110/80 |

## DIFFERENTIAL DIAGNOSIS OF HEART MURMURS

1. Serious heart disease *does* occur without a murmur. Myocarditis is then more likely than a congenital lesion
2. Rapid heart rate may obscure abnormal heart sounds and murmurs
3. Venous hums are often continuous and subclavicular. If heard on the left, may be confused with a PDA. Turning the head or lying down alters a hum but not a ductus murmur
4. Innocent murmurs
   - (i) Asymptomatic
   - (ii) No thrill
   - (iii) Localized to the left sternal border and apex
   - (iv) Short and musical, mid-systolic and grade 3/6 or less
   - (v) Varies with sitting up and lying down, often disappears on lying
5. Third heart sound is physiological, in early diastole, at the apex

## IMPORTANT PATHOLOGICAL FINDINGS

1. First sound
   An ejection click follows immediately after it in poststenotic dilatation of the pulmonary artery or aorta
2. Second sound
   (a) Loud in pulmonary hypertension
   (b) Soft and apparently single in pulmonary stenosis
   (c) Fixed split on breathing in/out in atrial septal defect
3. Murmurs
   Ejection systolic: increased flow, e.g. ASD secundum type or stenosis of pulmonary or aortic valve
   Pansystolic:   (i) shunt from higher to lower pressure, e.g. ventricular septal defect (VSD), atrial septal defect primum (ASD), patent ductus arteriosus (PDA)
              (ii) regurgitant, e.g. mitral incompetence
   Diastolic: early    = *regurgitant* incompetent aortic valve or pulmonary valve
          middle = *increased flow* from shunts (VSD, ASD, PDA) across normal valves
          late    = *obstructed flow* across a 'tight' tricuspid or mitral valve

*Continuous*
1. Patent ductus arteriosus (unusual in infancy, usually systolic)
2. Combinations AS and AI, MI and AI, VSD and AI
3. Coarctation of the aorta (due to collaterals, best heard over the back, in child over 5 years old)
4. Venous hum disappears on lying down, applying pressure on neck veins, or Valsva manoeuvre

## CONGENITAL HEART DISEASE

Frequency of congenital heart defects is 6 in 1000 children.
Relative frequency: VSD 30%, PDA 15%, others <10% each.

Acyanotic congenital heart disease — shunts*

| | Age-specific symptoms | Clinical signs of note |
|---|---|---|
| Patent ductus arteriosus (15%) | *Premature:* recurrent apnoea, persistent RDS, CCF *Infant:* 'chesty', FTT, CCF *Adult:* breathless, cyanosis, SBE | *Pulse:* bounding *Thrill:* 'to and fro' left infraclavicular area *Murmurs:* pansystolic in infancy becoming continuous and 'machinery' like ± mid-diastolic flow murmur from mitral valve at apex |
| Ventricular septal defect (30%) | *3 months: l*arge VSD — reduced pulmonary vascular resistance causes acute CCF ± cyanosis *Infant:* moderate VSD — 'chesty', FTT, CCF *Child:* small VSD asymptomatic, risk of SBE | *Pulse:* normal, or weak and rapid *Apex:* thrusting, laterally displaced *Thrill:* lower left sternal edge *Heart sounds:* 2nd is widely split, from increased filling of right ventricle *Murmurs:* harsh pansystolic ± mid-diastolic mitral flow at apex |
| Atrial septal defect: Ostium secundum (8%) | *Child:* asymptomatic *Adult:* breathless from pulmonary hypertension | *Pulse:* normal, no thrill *Heart sounds:* wide fixed split of 2nd sound from conduction delay (right bundle branch block) *Murmurs:* mid-systolic at 2nd left interspace ± mid-diastolic tricuspid flow at lower right sternal edge |
| Ostium primum (atrio-ventricular septal defect) (3%) | *Infant:* 'chesty', FTT, CCF *Child:* progressive cyanosis as shunt reverses from the pulmonary hypertension. Occurs in 40% of Down's | As for secundum + if mitral valve is cleft (common) *Thrill:* left sternal edge *Murmurs:* apical pansystolic is mitral valve incompetence |

*NB: chest X-ray in all but the mildest cases shows varying degrees of cardiac enlargement, pulmonary plethora and prominent pulmonary vessels.

Acyanotic congenital heart disease — obstructive

|  | Age-specific symptoms | Clinical signs of note |
|---|---|---|
| Aortic stenosis (various causes) (5%) | Infant:<br>(i) valvular: CCF if a severe stenosis<br>(ii) supravalvular: asymptomatic, unusual face, retarded development ↑Ca$^{2+}$ (William's syndrome)<br>Child & adult: valve/ obstructive cardiomyopathy — dizzy, angina, sudden death | Pulse: small volume, 'plateau'<br>Apex: thrust<br>Thrill: left sternal edge radiating up to the neck<br>Heart sounds: soft 2nd aortic part, the usual split may be reversed (i.e. ↑on expiration)<br>Murmurs: ejection systolic radiating to the neck |
| Coarctation of the aorta (6%) | Infant: breathless, CCF (VSD often present)<br>Child & adult: asymptomatic, rarely ruptured berry aneurysm, SBE | Differential cyanosis in neonates, i.e. pink above the ductus, blue below<br>Pulse: absent/weak/delayed femorals, elevated BP in upper limbs; hyperdynamic neck pulsations<br>Apex: thrusting<br>Murmur: ejection systolic radiates through to the back |
| Pulmonary stenosis (8%) | Infant: if severe, acute CCF ± cyanosis due to right to left shunt via foramen ovale; otherwise asymptomatic in children<br>Adult: CCF, arrhythmias | Jugular venous pulse: large 'a' wave; right ventricular heave<br>Thrill: 2nd left interspace<br>Heart sounds: soft 2nd<br>Murmurs: ejection click, then systolic ejection in 2nd interspace |
| Hypoplastic left heart | Few days old (2–6): CCF, pale, severe acidosis, simulates sepsis or an inborn error | Shock, low BP, death in days |

Cyanotic congenital heart disease

| | Age-specific symptoms | Specific signs |
|---|---|---|
| Transposition of the great arteries (4%) | Cyanosis from birth or shortly after, proportional to shunt through foramen ovale, ductus arteriosus or VSD. Breathless, CCF | Cyanosis: persists in 100% oxygen, which may even cause the cyanosis to worsen by causing closure of the ductus (= ductus dependent) Heart sounds: single Murmurs: often absent Chest X-ray*: 'egg on side' heart shape |
| Fallot's tetralogy (pulmonary infundibular stenosis, VSD, right ventricle hypertrophies, aorta overrides) (5%) | Infant: progressively deeper cyanosis, weeks or few months old. Cyanotic 'spells' from infundibular spasm Childhood: 'squatting' after exertion, SBE, cerebral abscesses, polycythemia | Colour: cyanosis, clubbing Palpation: right ventricular heave Heart sounds: single 2nd Murmurs: ejection systolic at 3rd left interspace Chest X-ray*: 'boot shaped' heart |
| Eisenmenger syndrome of irreversible pulmonary hypertension | Infant or child with VSD, transposition of the great arteries, PDA, or commonly an atrioventricular canal in Down's syndrome. Torrential flow of blood through lungs causes the pulmonary vessels to thicken, irreversibly | Palpation: right parasternal (ventricular) heave and the pulmonary valve closing Heart sounds: loud pulmonary 2nd Murmurs: ejection systolic ± early diastolic from pulmonary regurgitation |

*Classical finding present in only a half of cases.

CCF = congestive cardiac failure; FTT = failure to thrive; RDS = respiratory distress syndrome; SBE = subacute bacterial endocarditis; VSD = ventricular septal defect; PDA = patent ductus arteriosus.

## CAUSES OF SINUS TACHYCARDIA

Common
1. Fever
2. Anaemia
3. Drugs: theophylline, β sympathomimetics
4. Hypovolaemia

*Uncommon*
5. Congestive cardiac failure
*Rare*
6. Hyperthyroidism
7. Kawasaki disease

## CAUSES OF SINUS BRADYCARDIA

*Common*
1. Physiological
2. Premature
*Uncommon*
3. Raised intracranial pressure
4. Hypoxaemia
*Rare*
5. Digoxin (as now rarely used except in acute myocarditis and endocardial fibroelastosis)
6. Hypothyroidism

## CAUSES OF CARDIAC FAILURE

*Common*
1. Stress: fever, hypoxia, infection, acidosis, hypoglycaemia
2. Anaemia, especially prematures, polycythemia
3. Fluid overload
4. Cardiac
    (i) Neonatal
        (a) Volume overload: PDA
        *Uncommon*
        (b) Pressure overload: hypoplastic left heart, coarctation
        (c) Pump failure = myocarditis: coxsackie B
        (d) Arrhythmia: complete heart block
    (ii) Infancy
        *Common*
        (a) Volume overload as pulmonary vascular resistance falls in the first weeks of life: VSD
        (b) Pressure overload: pulmonary hypertension, pulmonary stenosis
        *Uncommon*
        (c) Myocarditis: endocardial fibroelastosis, infection, e.g. mumps, Echo, Kawasaki disease
        (d) Arrhythmia: paroxysmal supraventricular tachycardia
    (iii) Child: systemic hypertension, pulmonary hypertension, bacterial endocarditis, myocarditis
*Rare*
5. Thyrotoxicosis

## CAUSES OF CYANOSIS

*Common*
1. Depression of central nervous system: drugs, trauma, asphyxia
2. Seizures
3. Respiratory disease
4. Stress: septicaemia, hypoglycaemia, adrenal crisis, Reye's syndrome

*Less common*
5. Polycythaemia in the newborn
6. Cardiac: *any age* — arrhythmias, myocarditis
   (i) *Neonate:* transposition of the great arteries (TGA), persistent fetal circulation, atresia or stenosis of the pulmonary or tricuspid valves
   (ii) *Infant:* Fallot's tetralogy, tricuspid atresia
   (iii) *Child:* Pulmonary hypertension — Eisenmenger's syndrome

## CAUSES OF RAISED BLOOD PRESSURE

**Acute**
1. Renal: acute glomerulonephritis, trauma
2. Burns
3. CNS: infection, space occupation
4. Haemolytic uraemic syndrome

**Chronic**
1. Renal: infected, scarred, obstructed and congenitally abnormal kidneys, tumours
2. Vascular: renal artery stenosis, coarctation of the aorta
3. Corticosteroids (including Cushing's syndrome)

## CAUSES OF CHEST PAIN

*Very common*
1. Non-organic: idiopathic, anxiety related, hyperventilation
2. Musculoskeletal: trauma, exercise, costochondritis
   (Uncommon: shingles (Herpes zoster))
*Common*
3. Chest: asthma, pneumonia, sickle cell 'chest syndrome', pneumothorax
*Uncommon*
4. Oesophagitis
*Rare*
5. Cardiac: pericarditis, endocarditis

## CLINICAL CHARACTERISTICS OF SYSTEMIC JUVENILE CHRONIC ARTHRITIS (STILL'S DISEASE), RHEUMATIC FEVER AND HENOCH-SCHÖNLEIN (ANAPHYLACTOID) PURPURA

|  | Still's | Rheumatic fever | Henoch-Schönlein |
|---|---|---|---|
| Cause | Autoimmune | βHS | βHS, viral, allergy |
| Age | 1–5 years | 4–7 years | >1 year, peak at 5 years |
| Fever | Diurnal/any pattern | Sustained | Normal/raised |
| Rash | Maculopapular | Erythema marginatum | Urticarial/purpuric |
| Joints | Neck, knee, hip, foot, hand | Wrist, elbow, knee, ankle | Wrist, ankle, knee |
| RES | Glands, hepato-splenomegaly | Liver ++ if in heart failure | No enlargement |
| Heart | Pericarditis | Pericarditis and carditis | No involvement |
| Urine | Normal | Normal | Haematuria |
| Abdomen | Occasional pain | Normal | Acute pain common |
| Duration | Months | Days < weeks | Days > weeks |

βHS = β–haemolytic streptococcus; RES = Reticulo-endothelial system

## KAWASAKI DISEASE: CRITERIA FOR DIAGNOSIS

*Five features (atypically three or more) of the following are needed for diagnosis:*
1. Temperature for 5 or more days
2. Rash, erythematous, macular or multiforme
3. Oedema of hands and feet, peeling of the skin of fingertips
4. Conjunctivitis, bilateral
5. Lips dry, cracked, peeling, erythematous; strawberry tongue; pharyngeal erythema
6. Cervical lymphadenopathy, non-suppurative

## RADIOLOGICAL FEATURES TO LOOK FOR

### Normal
1. Cardiothoracic ratio (CTR) of 0.50 or less, except between 12 and 18 months, when the upper limit is 0.55
2. Thymus shadow may give impression of cardiomegaly, but sail shape or wave sign helps to discriminate. In cyanotic conditions the thymus rapidly involutes

### Changes in pulmonary blood flow (PBF)
1. Cyanotic congenital heart disease

| *Reduced PBF* | *Increased PBF* |
|---|---|
| Fallot's tetralogy | Transposition of great arteries |
| Pulmonary atresia | Truncus arteriosus |

2. Acyanotic congenital heart disease

| *Normal PBF* | *Increased PBF* | *Reduced PBF* |
|---|---|---|
| Coarctation | Atrial septal defect | Pulmonary stenosis |
| Aortic stenosis | Ventricular septal defect | Pulmonary |
|  | Patent ductus arteriosus | hypertension |

### Cardiomegaly (CTR >0.5)
*Common*
1. Congestive cardiac failure
*Uncommon*
2. Pericardial effusion
3. Myocarditis
4. Cardiomyopathy
5. Complete heart block

# Gastroenterology

## CAUSES OF UMBILICAL HERNIA

*Common*
1. Physiological, especially African
2. Premature
*Uncommon/rare*
3. Down's syndrome
4. Hypothyroidism
5. Mucopolysaccharidoses

## CAUSES OF INGUINAL SWELLINGS

1. Enlarged lymph glands
2. Inguinal hernia
3. Hydrocoele (inguinal hernia may be associated with it)
4. Undescended testis

## CAUSES OF GINGIVOSTOMATITIS

*Common*
1. Infection
    (i) Viruses: primary herpes simplex, Coxsackie A (herpangina; hand, foot and mouth disease)
    (ii) Bacteria: streptococcus (rarely diphtheria, Vincent's angina)
    (iii) Fungal: monilia (secondary to antibiotics, bottle feeding, prematurity, HIV, rare immune deficiency syndromes)
2. Aphthous ulcers: alone or with coeliac disease
3. Local reaction: mouth washes, cheek biting
4. Drugs and poisons: phenytoin, oral contraceptives, pregnancy
*Uncommon*
5. Kawasaki disease (p 54)
6. Stevens–Johnson syndrome

## CAUSES OF HAEMATEMESIS

*NB: Exclude colourings (beetroot, food dyes) as a cause first.*

*Common*
1. Swallowed blood
   (i) Neonate: maternal, at birth or cracked nipple
   (ii) Epistaxis
2. Vomiting repeatedly, acute gastritis
*Less common*
3. Ulceration
   (i) Hiatus hernia
   (ii) Drugs: aspirin, iron poisoning
   (iii) Peptic ulcer
   (iv) Foreign body
4. Munchausen by proxy (factitious bleeding)
*Rare but important*
5. Oesophageal varices, bleeding disorders, vascular
   malformations, e.g. haemangioma

## CLINICAL FEATURES OF HIATUS HERNIA VERSUS PYLORIC STENOSIS

|  | Hiatus hernia | Pyloric stenosis |
|---|---|---|
| Age at onset | First week | 2–6 weeks |
| Sex | Males = females | Firstborn males (M:F = 5:1) |
| Family history | — | In 20% |
| Vomiting | Continuous, wells up, fresh/altered blood if ulceration present; no bile | Forceful, soon after feeds; altered blood occasionally; no bile |
| Nutrition | Slowly progressive failure to thrive | Acute weight loss, dehydration; metabolic alkalosis; sodium ion depletion |
| Associated symptoms (aspiration) | Cyanotic episodes, wheeze; pyloric mass palpable; palor (anaemia) | Visible peristalsis or pneumonia |
| Stools | Occasionally constipated, altered blood | Starvation stools/ constipated |

*N.B. Feeding mismanagement and urinary infections share many of these symptoms and signs.*

## CAUSES OF VOMITING

*Common*
1. Non-organic
   (i) Infants: tension between mother and infant, domestic stress, overfeeding, posseting (rarely: rumination)
   (ii) Toddler: food refusal may be a battle for control with carers
   (iii) Children: self-induced, overeating
   (iv) Adolescents: anorexia nervosa/bulimia nervosa
2. Infection: gastroenteritis or as parenteral response to urine infection, otitis media, etc.
3. Cough: pertussis, asthma

*Less common*
4. Gastrointestinal disorders
   (i) Medical: hiatus hernia, food allergies (cow's milk protein intolerance), coeliac disease
   (ii) Surgical: pyloric stenosis, acute obstruction, appendicitis; repeated episodes may occur in malrotation
5. Migraine, cyclical vomiting
6. Medication: emetics, valproate, flucloxacillin

*Uncommon but important*
7. Metabolic: diabetes mellitus, uraemia, congenital adrenal hyperplasia
8. Raised intracranial pressure

### Projectile vomiting

*Common*
1. Urinary tract infection
2. Pyloric stenosis
3. Cow's milk protein intolerance

*Uncommon*
4. Obstruction: duodenal stenosis or atresia, malrotation of the bowel
5. Raised intracranial pressure

*Rare*
6. Duodenal ulcer, adrenal insufficiency due to inborn error

## CAUSES OF ABDOMINAL DISTENSION

### Neonatal
See p16.

### Infancy and childhood

*Common*
1. Obesity
2. Air swallowing: feeding, habit is rare tracheo-oesophageal fistula

3. Intestinal
   (i) Peritonitis, paralytic ileus, acute obstruction
   (ii) Dysentery
   (iii) Faecal impaction
   *Uncommon*
   (i) Malabsorption: coeliac disease, meconium ileus equivalent
      in cystic fibrosis
   (ii) Inflammatory bowel disease: Crohn's, ulcerative colitis
   *Rare but important:* Hirschsprung's disease
4. Abdominal masses: renal, hepatosplenomegaly, rarely
   malignancies
*Uncommon*
5. Ascites: cardiac, malnutrition, nephrotic, nephritic, malignant,
   cirrhotic

## CAUSES OF ACUTE ABDOMINAL PAIN

**Medical**
Exclude coughing and associated straining of rectus abdominus.
*Common*
1. Infection: gastroenteritis, 'mesenteric adenitis', lower lobe
   pneumonia, urinary tract infection, acute hepatitis
2. Constipation
*Uncommon*
3. Henoch-Schönlein (anaphylactoid) purpura
4. Acute nephritis
*Rare but important*
5. Miscellaneous, e.g. diabetes mellitus, sickle cell crisis, Kawasaki
   disease

**Surgical**
*Common*
1. Acute appendicitis
2. Obstruction: intussusception, strangulated inguinal hernia,
   volvulus
*Uncommon*
3. Renal: hydronephrosis, colic
4. Gynaecological/testicular: torsion of ovary or testis, pelvic
   inflammatory disease, ectopic pregnancy

## CAUSES OF RECURRENT ABDOMINAL PAIN

**Definition**
Three discrete episodes of abdominal pain in a 3 month period,
interfering with regular activities and school attendance; it affects
10% of school children.

*Common*
1. Migrainous or psychological stress in 95%
*Less common*
2. Mesenteric adenitis
3. Constipation
4. Food allergy, lactose intolerance
*Uncommon*
5. GIT: worms, oesophagitis, irritable bowel syndrome, Crohn's disease, ulcerative colitis, peptic ulcer
6. Renal: hydronephrosis, recurrent pyelonephritis, calculi

## CLINICAL FEATURES OF APPENDICITIS VERSUS MESENTERIC ADENITIS

|  | *Appendicitis* | *Mesenteric adenitis* |
| --- | --- | --- |
| Recurrence | — | Previous episodes common |
| Upper respiratory tract infection | Maybe | Within 24 hours, cervical glands +/++ |
| Temperature and appearance | Usually 38°C (in preschool up to 40°C), ill, becomes toxic | 39–40°C common, flushed |
| Vomiting | Frequent | Unusual |
| Abdominal tenderness, guarding | Marked, usually very distressed, localized to right side, young child pushes hand away ++ | Vague, generalized, periumbilical, often comes and goes |
| Rectal examination | Localized tenderness on right | No localized tenderness |

## CAUSES OF CARBOHYDRATE MALABSORPTION

*Confirmation:* Solid stool is not suitable so collection is made by placing the baby on plastic and the stool–water: water mix of 1:2 is tested using Clinitest. >0.5% sugar is a positive result.

*Common*
1. Secondary disaccharidase deficiency, usually lactase
      (i) Infective gastroenteritis, giardiasis
      (ii) Cow's milk protein intolerance

## CAUSES OF ACUTE DIARRHOEA

*Common*
1. Infection: rota and enterovirus, *Escherichia coli*, shigella, salmonella, campylobacter, giardia, amoeba, yersinia
2. Food poisoning toxins: staphylococcal
3. Parenteral response to infection, e.g. pneumonia, otitis media, etc.
4. Starvation stools (mucousy, watery and green)

*Less common*
5. Surgical: pelvic appendicitis, Hirschsprung's disease (as colitis)
6. Drugs: laxatives, directly or via breast milk, antibiotics

## CAUSES OF CHRONIC DIARRHOEA

*Common*
1. Normal growth, loose or semiformed stools
    (i) Chronic non-specific toddler's diarrhoea
    (ii) Constipation with overflow
    (iii) Laxative abuse as a form of Munchausen by proxy, or in bulimia nervosa in an older child

*Less common*
2. Failure to gain weight, or actual weight loss, and persistent loose watery stools for more than 2 weeks
    (i) Enteric infections: see above; note that immunodeficiency may be present
    (ii) Postenteric infection: lactose and cow's milk protein intolerance, transient gluten enteropathy
    (iii) Inflammatory bowel disease: food allergies, ulcerative colitis, Crohn's disease
    (iv) Malabsorption: coeliac disease, cystic fibrosis

## CHARACTERISTICS OF CYSTIC FIBROSIS AND COELIAC DISEASE

| | Cystic fibrosis | Coeliac (untreated) |
|---|---|---|
| **Newborn** | Meconium ileus | — |
| **Infant** | Failure to thrive from birth; recurrent pneumonia (*S. aureus* or *Pseudomonas* almost diagnostic) | Failure to thrive from introduction of gluten, usually at 3–4 months old |
| 1. Stools | Often abnormal from birth, diarrhoeal, very smelly, oily like melted butter | Normal until gluten introduced; become pale and bulky; not oily |
| 2. Appetite | Voracious | Poor |
| 3. Chest | 'Bronchitis' frequent, i.e. recurrent bronchopneumonia | Normal |
| 4. Social | Lively | Withdrawn, 'difficult' |
| 5. Others | Rectal prolapse, salty taste to skin, heat exhaustion | Anaemia, rickets, long eyelashes |
| **Child** As above plus: | | |
| 1. Height | Relatively preserved | Short |
| 2. Puberty | Delayed, males sterile | Delayed, amenorrhoea common in girls |
| 3. Abdomen | Meconium ileus equivalent; biliary cirrhosis and portal hypertension cause enlarged spleen and oesophageal varices | Distended, liver edge not palpable, wasted buttocks |
| 4. Others | Cor pulmonale; nasal polyps; diabetes mellitus | School failure from lethargy |
| **Screening** | Neonatal blood trypsin level elevated (Guthrie card may be used) | Antibodies to gliadin, antireticulin, antiendomysium (also used to monitor dietary compliance) |
| **Diagnosis** | Sweat sodium 70 mmol/l or more on at least 100 mg of sweat | Villous atrophy, heals on diet, relapses on normal diet, seen on jejunal biopsies |

## CAUSES OF CONSTIPATION

*Common*
1. Familial, habit, lack of fibre
2. Voluntary: encopresis, anal fissure
3. Starvation, dehydration
*Uncommon*
4. Obstruction, paralytic ileus
5. Neurological: hypotonia, cerebral palsy, mental retardation
*Rare*
6. Metabolic: hypothyroidism

## CAUSES OF COLORECTAL BLEEDING (after the neonatal period)

NB: (i) Exclude coloured drinks or beetroot as the cause, by history.
    (ii) Fresh bleeding is usually large bowel, malaena may be from a more proximal site higher up
*Common*
1. Constipation, anal fissure
2. Dysentery and salmonellosis
*Uncommon*
3. Intussusception
4. Henoch-Schönlein anaphylactoid purpura
5. Cow's milk protein intolerance
6. Acid ulceration: hiatus hernia, peptic ulcer, Meckel's diverticulum
7. Swallowed blood and bleeding diathesis
8. Ulcerative colitis, Crohn's disease
9. Munchausen by proxy (may be colouring/dye/animal or menstrual blood)

## CAUSES OF HEPATOSPLENOMEGALY

*Common*
1. Infection: hepatitis A and B, infectious mononucleosis, malaria, septicaemia, HIV
*Uncommon*
2. Haematological: mainly splenic enlargement in spherocytosis, sickle cell, severe iron deficiency anaemia, thrombocytopenia
3. Congestive cardiac failure, mainly liver enlargement
4. Malignancy: leukaemia, lymphoma, secondary deposits in the liver, e.g. neuroblastoma
*Rare*
5. Miscellaneous: portal hypertension, storage disorders (e.g. Gaucher's)

## CAUSES OF JAUNDICE IN INFANTS AND CHILDREN

**Neonates** See p12.

**Unconjugated ('indirect' reading hyperbilirubinaemia)**
1. Haemolytic: spherocytosis, sickle cell, thalassaemia, glucose-6-phosphatase deficiency
2. Metabolic: Gilbert's disease (dominantly inherited diminished ability of uptake of bilirubin by liver cells)

**Conjugated ('direct') bilirubin >25 μmol/l (1.5 mg/100 ml)**
1. Infection: hepatitis A and B, urinary infection, malaria
2. Drugs, e.g. paracetamol poisoning, valproate risk in under 2 year olds
3. Metabolic, e.g. Reye's syndrome associated with aspirin taken during influenza or chicken pox
*Rare but important*
4. Biliary obstruction: biliary atresia in infancy
5. Chronic inflammatory disease, e.g. chronic active hepatitis in older children

# Haematology

## NORMAL CHANGES IN HAEMATOLOGY

Birth:     Haemoglobin (Hb) 19 g/dl at term, 16 g/dl in premature infants
Lymphocytes predominate from the end of the first week of life through to late childhood
HbF (fetal haemoglobin) is more than 50% of total Hb
1st year:  Hb falls to its lowest level at about 2 months, and thereafter averages 11 g/dl. HbF is 5% of total at 6 months
Childhood: 12 g/dl

## CAUSES OF ANAEMIA

1. Decreased production, especially iron deficiency anaemia
2. Increased destruction (haemolysis)
3. Blood loss

## CAUSES OF HYPOCHROMIC (IRON DEFICIENCY) ANAEMIA

*Common*
1. Nutritional
   (i) Prolonged milk feeding and foods containing inadequate iron
   (ii) Malnutrition
2. Prematurity
   (i) 'Early anaemia' at 4–6 weeks: dilutional owing to rapid growth and therefore normochromic
   (ii) Inadequate iron stores: 'late anaemia' at 8–12 weeks (a macrocytic anaemia due to folic acid or vitamin E deficiency can also occur within this time period)
3. Chronic infection, e.g. urinary tract infection (more often presents as *normochromic* anaemia)
4. Cow's milk protein intolerance

*Uncommon*
5. Peptic ulceration, e.g. hiatus hernia, Meckel's diverticulum causing loss of iron via bleeding
6. Malabsorption, e.g. coeliac disease

## CAUSES OF HAEMOLYTIC ANAEMIA, BY AGE AT PRESENTATION

**Neonatal**
1. Acquired
   (i) Immune: Rhesus, ABO
   (ii) Infection: congenital (TORCH), and acquired
2. Genetic
   (i) Enzyme deficiency, e.g. glucose-6-phosphate dehydrogenase deficiency (G6PD) is sex linked; Mediterranean, Asian and males of African origin mainly affected. Haemolysis is spontaneous in newborn, later episodes precipitated by drugs, fava beans and sepsis
   (ii) Spherocytosis: deficiency of spectrin in the RBC membrane, autosomal dominant, large spleen, jaundice and anaemia, gall stones in adults

**Infancy**
1. Infection, acute, e.g. septicaemia, malaria. Meningococcaemia may cause disseminated intravascular coagulation
2. Genetic: sickle cell disease and thalassaemia both become manifest from 6 months as HbF production falls
3. Haemolytic–uraemic syndrome

**Childhood**
1. Acquired
   (i) Infection, acute: see above
   (ii) Autoimmune Coombs' positive anaemia after infections, e.g. mycoplasma, viral, also idiopathic, or may be drug induced
   (iii) Drugs, e.g. penicillin, sulpha, nitrofurantoin
2. Genetic, e.g. sickle cell, thalassaemia, spherocytosis, G6PD

## CAUSES OF ACUTE AND CHRONIC BLOOD LOSS

Perinatal: see p 13.
1. Epistaxis
2. Trauma
3. Ulceration: hiatus hernia, peptic ulcer, Meckel's diverticulum
4. Thrombocytopenia, e.g. idiopathic thrombocytopenia, leukaemia
5. Coagulation disorder, e.g. vitamin K deficiency, haemophilia

## CAUSES OF A LOW MEAN CORPUSCULAR VOLUME (MCV)

1. Iron deficiency anaemia
2. Thalassaemia trait — normal red cell count and normal mean corpuscular haemoglobin concentration (MCHC), *low* mean corpuscular haemoglobin (MCH)
3. Lead poisoning

**Causes of clinical characteristics of bleeds from vascular or platelet defect and coagulation defect**

| Haemostasis factors | Examples of causes | Clinical |
|---|---|---|
| 1. Vascular integrity | Venous obstruction, e.g. vomiting, coughing, Henoch–Schönlein purpura; infections, e.g. meningococcaemia | (i) Petechiae, purpura, echymoses<br>(ii) Epistaxis, GI bleeds, menorrhagia<br>(iii) Bleeds stop on local pressure |
| 2. Platelets (<100 × 10⁹/l) | (i) Consumed: shock, septicaemia<br>(ii) Less produced: idiopathic thrombocytopenia, replaced by tumour tissue/leukaemia cells<br>(iii) Function: von Willebrand disease | |
| 3. Coagulation | (i) Alone: haemophilia<br>(ii) Combined: disseminated intravascular coagulation (+platelets consumed) | (i) Cut → *delayed* onset of bleed<br>(ii) *Deep* bleeds, single site, e.g. joint, muscle; haematuria<br>(iii) Local pressure fails to stop bleeding |

## CAUSES OF BRUISING

1. Trauma, accidental and non-accidental
2. Vascular (see above) ⎫
3. Platelets (see above) ⎬ either may present as purpura
4. Coagulation defects
    (i) Haemorrhagic disease of the newborn (vitamin K dependent factors — prothrombin, VII, IX, X)
    (ii) Consumption: shock, asphyxia, meningococcaemia
    (iii) Inherited: sex linked factor deficiencies VIII, IX = haemophilia (VIII), Christmas disease (IX)

# Oncology

## RELATIVE FREQUENCY OF CHILDHOOD MALIGNANCIES

1. Acute lymphoblastic leukaemia (ALL) 30%
2. Brain tumours 20%
3. Lymphoma 15%

## COMMON AGE AT PRESENTATION OF MALIGNANCIES

| | |
|---|---|
| Infancy: | Neuroblastoma |
| 2–4 years: | ALL |
| | Wilms' tumour of kidney |
| 7 years: | Lymphoma (non-Hodgkin) |
| >10 years: | Ewing's sarcoma of bone |

## CAUSES OF HIGH WHITE CELL COUNT (WBC) (lymphocytes excessively high)

1. Glandular fever, cytomegalovirus (both have atypical lymphocytes)
2. Pertussis (cough is obvious)
3. Still's disease (p 54) (may be difficult to differentiate clinically from leukaemia)
4. Leukaemia

## CONDITIONS PRESENTING LIKE LEUKAEMIA

1. Anaemia (see p 65)
2. Glandular fever
3. Oral infection, e.g. herpes stomatitis
4. Idiopathic thrombocytopenia
5. Bone pains from Still's disease, neuroblastoma

## CHARACTERISTICS OF CEREBRAL TUMOURS

Most (70%) are infratentorial in the posterior fossa and symptoms are those of:
1. Raised intracranial pressure, e.g. headache and vomiting
2. Ataxia due to cerebellar involvement. May be unilateral or bilateral depending on site of tumour
3. Cranial nerve palsies due to infiltration and as false localizing signs from raised intracranial pressure (VIth cranial nerve)
4. Torticollis

Differential diagnosis of Wilms' tumour and abdominal neuroblastoma

|  | Wilms' tumour | Neuroblastoma |
| --- | --- | --- |
| Age (years) | <5 | <2 |
| Health | Well | Usually ill |
| Clinical | Swollen abdomen | Pale, weight loss and bone pain common |
| Mass | Lobulated, firm | Irregular edge, 'craggy' |
| Crosses midline | Rare | Common |
| Bilateral | Rare | Occasional |
| IVP pelvis | Grossly distorted | Pushed down, by mass above |
| Metastases (common sites) | Lungs | Bone (orbits) |

# Immunology, common infectious diseases and vaccinations

## NORMAL DEVELOPMENT OF IMMUNE SYSTEM

### Fetal

Immunoglobulins of G class pass from mother to baby and are not only responsible for protecting baby but also cause disease, e.g. rhesus incompatability.

### Newborn

Maternal origin and levels of immunoglobulin G (IgA and IgM low), falling progressively to very low level by 3 months.

Neutrophils are active but not yet good at fighting infection and thus babies are at increased risk of bacterial infection.

Lymphocyte function (B and T cell) not well developed, manifest by frequent superficial fungal (candida) infection and greater susceptibility to herpes simplex virus.

Thymus is large and easily seen on X-ray. It shrinks rapidly in stress or cyanotic congenital heart disease.

### Infant

Breast feeding protects via IgA, lactoferrin, interferon, lysozyme, and maternal macrophages in the milk. Progressive rise in the infant's own immunoglobulins and cellular immunity to near normal by 6 months, slow increase to adult levels in the first 5 years of life.

## CAUSES OF RECURRENT INFECTION

1. Normal development of immunity
2. Socioeconomic, and infants who are bottle fed (hygiene) or whose parents smoke
3. Secondary to disease:
   (i) Malnutrition
   (ii) HIV
   (iii) Steroids, other drugs, i.e. side effect of treatment
   (iv) Predisposing disorder, e.g. cystic fibrosis; structural abnormality, e.g. cleft palate and otitis media, splenectomy and septicaemia
   (v) Protein losing, e.g. nephrotic syndrome
4. Primary immune deficiency of immunoglobulins, white cells or complement systems

### Allergy

A state of altered reactivity, i.e. a change in the host's response after exposure to a 'foreign' (allergenic) substance, e.g. drugs, environmental or host's body constituents.

| Type and clinical onset | Reaction | Examples |
|---|---|---|
| 1. Anaphylactic or reagin-dependent *Onset:* immediate | Reaginic antibody (IgE) bound to tissue cells (e.g. mast cells) on contact with an antigen (e.g. pollen), release of histamine, bradykinin, etc | (i) Anaphylaxis<br>(ii) Hay fever, asthma<br>(iii) Urticaria<br>(iv) Food allergies<br>(v) Drug allergies |
| 2. Cytotoxic *Onset:* minutes to hours | Circulating antibody (IgG or IgM) reacts with antigen bound to cell surface, usually in presence of complement cell damage | (i) Drug Induced<br>(ii) Rhesus, ABO iso-immunization<br>(iii) Blood transfusion |
| 3. Circulating immune complexes *Onset:* hours to days | Freely circulating antigen and antibody combine in presence of complement to form microprecipitates, and damage to small blood vessels | (i) Post streptococal nephritis<br>(ii) Serum sickness<br>(iii) Erythema multiforme, the Arthus phenomenon, e.g. to sulphonamides |
| 4. Cell-mediated, or delayed hypersensitivity *Onset:* days | Sensitized lymphocytes react with an antigen deposited at a local site and release lymphokines such as mitogenic factor | (i) Eczema<br>(ii) Contact dermatitis<br>(iii) Tuberculin tests<br>(iv) Graft versus host |

## SOME IMPORTANT INFECTIOUS DISEASES

| Disease | Incubation (days) | Characteristics and complications | Communicability |
|---|---|---|---|
| Chicken pox | 14 (7–21) | Vesicles spread down face, trunk, proximal parts of limbs. Pneumonia, ataxia | −2 to +7 days from start of rash until spots crusted (dry) |
| Diphtheria | 3 (1–6) | Grey–white membrane in nose, throat, 'toxic', myocarditis, bulbar palsy | 4 weeks or negative swabs ×2 |
| Enteric bacteria (salmonella, etc., *E. coli*) | 3–23 | 3 major patterns: 1. Diarrhoea 2. Septicaemia 3. Cholera like | Until asymptomatic and 3 negative stools |
| Fifth, or slapped cheek, disease | 4–14 | Bright spots on cheeks, coalesce to look like a 'slap'; fine rash to body | 1 week, not apparent under 2 years old |
| Glandular fever | 14–56 | Sore throat, fever, lethargy, glands+++, hepatosplenomegaly, encephalitis, polyneuritis | 3 months, avoid salivary contact (cups, kissing) |
| Infectious hepatitis | 15–40 | Anicteric, itchy, anorexic; to icteric, pale stools, dark urine. Tender liver/ abdomen mimics appendicitis | 7 days minimum |
| Measles | 10 (7–24) | 'Cold', photophobia, Koplik's spots, fever; then red rash (face to trunk), conjunctivitis, otitis media, pneumonia, encephalitis day 5–10 of illness | From 'cold' to 7 days after rash appears |
| Mumps | 17 (14–28) | Fever, sore throat, pain on chewing, furred tongue, swollen parotid. Meningoencephalitis. Rarely orchitis, pancreatitis in children | −9 to +9 days after onset of swelling or when swelling goes |

## SOME IMPORTANT INFECTIOUS DISEASES (contd.)

| Disease | Incubation (days) | Characteristics and complications | Communicability |
|---------|-------------------|-----------------------------------|-----------------|
| Pertussis | 10 (7–14) | Catarrhal for 1–2 weeks, then paroxysmal cough ± whoop 14–100 days. Recurs for up to 2 years. Death 1% if <6 months old | 5 weeks from onset of cough |
| Polio | 14 (7–21) | 'Cold', diarrhoea, muscle aches; after 7 days 'meningitic' and temperature rises again. Paralytic phase 3–7 days after onset of preparalytic meningitic phase. Spinal and bulbar forms | Until stool negative for virus, i.e. weeks |
| Roseola | (5–15) | Fever for 3–4 days, as temperature falls rose–pink papules appear on trunk, neck, arms for a day | |
| Rubella | 17 (14–19) | Mild 'cold' then rash (fine maculopapular), which fades from face as it spreads downwards, Thrombocytopenia 3 weeks after, arthritis in adolescence, congenital infection in pregnancy | 7 days from onset of rash |
| Scarlet fever | 2–5 | Tonsillitis, red spots on palate, strawberry tongue, red face with circum-oral pallor, fine red rash spreads to whole of body by 2–3 days, may then shed fine skin scales. Arthritis, nephritis | 3 days from start of penicillin |

## IMMUNIZATION SCHEDULE

**Diphtheria-pertussis-tetanus (DPT), oral polio and *H. influenzae* b (Hib)**
At 2, 3 and 4 months old
School entry: omit pertussis, Hib
School leaving: omit pertussis, diphtheria, Hib

**Measles-mumps-rubella (MMR)**
12–18 months old

**BCG**
10–13 years if Heaf test negative

**Rubella**
10–14 years for girls who have not received MMR

**Special situations**
1. Prevention of vertical transmission of Hepatitis B from mothers who are carriers or recently infected
2. Neonatal BCG in UK in inner cities with high proportion of Asians
3. Pneumococcal vaccine for sickle cell disease, nephrotic syndrome, post splenectomy in children over 2 years old
4. Annual influenza vaccination for cystic fibrosis, severe asthma and diabetes sufferers

## CONTRAINDICATIONS TO PERTUSSIS IMMUNIZATION

**Absolute contraindications**
1. *Severe* local indurated swelling of most of upper arm circumference or lateral thigh following a previous injection
2. General reaction with temperature >39.4°C within 48 hours, persistent screaming >2 hours, unresponsiveness, anaphylaxis or convulsions within 72 hours

**Relative contraindications**
1. Cerebral damage documented in the neonatal period
2. Personal history of convulsions
3. First-degree relative with idiopathic epilepsy
   (For 1–3: Although chances of reactions may be higher in immunizing these children, they should still be protected as benefits outweigh the risks)

**General contraindications**
1. Acute febrile illness: delay vaccination for 1 week
2. Anaphylaxis following egg (give MMR vaccine in hospital) or specific antibiotic (traces of neomycin and kanamycin in mumps and MMR vaccine)
3. Immunodeficient or immunosupressed
   (i) Live vaccines are prohibited. Exception is MMR in HIV, and acute leukaemia in remission for >6 months
   (ii) Give specific immunoglobulin i.m. after exposure to measles, chickenpox. Parents must be aware of the need for treatment after contact.
   (iii) Measles vaccination is essential for siblings and close contacts
   (iv) Inactivated polio vaccine only, not live oral polio vaccine (OPV)

NB: Common parental misconceptions about contraindications include prematurity, heart disease and a family history of eczema or asthma.

## HUMAN IMMUNODEFICIENCY VIRUS (HIV)

### Mode of transmission and prognosis

1. Vertical by materno-fetal spread, prenatal, rarely by breast milk. 13% of infants become HIV positive. Of these, AIDS develops in a quarter by a year (of whom the majority die of HIV-related disease within that time), four-fifths by 4 years
2. Horizontal by infected blood or blood products (haemophiliacs)

### Presentation

| AIDS indicator diseases | Other HIV manifestations |
| --- | --- |
| Opportunistic infections | Persistent/recurrent oral candidiasis, parotitis |
| Severe recurrent bacterial infections | Persistent diarrhoea |
| Lipoid interstitial pneumonitis (LIP) | Persistent hepatosplenomegaly, lymphadenopathy |
| Severe failure to thrive | Severe/recurrent varicella |
| HIV encephalopathy (common at presentation) | |
| Malignancy (rare in childhood) | |

1. Infections, becoming recurrent:
   (i) Bacterial pneumonia, meningitis, recurrent otitis media, sinusitis
   (ii) Oral candidiasis, persistent and recurrent, and herpes stomatitis
   (iii) Acute interstitial pneumonitis = cough and dyspnoea, extensive infiltrates on X-ray. Due to *Pneumocystis pneumonia* (PCP) in 75%. Mortality is high. Other infections include TB, CMV, opportunistic infections
   (iv) Chronic lyphocytic interstitial pneumonitis (LIP), mean onset 14 months. Restrictive disease on respiratory function testing, proceeds to respiratory distress and hypoxia. Chest X-ray: hilar glands, lung infiltrates. Hypergammaglobulinaemia (>30 g/L)
   (iv) *Hycobacterium avium intracellulare* ('atypical'). High mortality
2. Failure to thrive, malabsorption. Poor appetite aggravated by the pain associated with oropharyngeal candidiasis
3. Non-specific. Lymphadenopathy, hepatosplenomegaly, eczematous skin rash, monilial nappy rash, persistent diarrhoea (75% initially present in this way)
4. Parotid gland swelling.
5. Encephalopathy (50%). Developmental delay or regression, pyramidal signs, ataxia, cortical atrophy

### Diagnosis

HIV antibody in first 18 months may be passively acquired from the mother. If the child develops signs or symptoms of disease before this time, the diagnosis can be made earlier.

Indicative of infection: polyclonal hypergammaglobulinaemia, and low CD4 (cluster determinant) lymphocyte counts.

Differential diagnosis: Primary immune disorders, cystic fibrosis, CNS degenerative disease.

# Renal disorders

## RENAL DISORDERS BY AGE AT PRESENTATION

### Neonate and infant
*Common*
1. Urinary tract infection (males >females)
*Uncommon*
2. Renal failure, e.g. Potter's renal agenesis syndrome, dysplasia, obstructive lesions, asphyxia
3. Haemolytic uraemic syndrome
*Rare*
4. Nephrogenic diabetes insipidus

### Toddlers and older
*Common*
1. Urinary tract infection (females >males). Ascending infection common, obstructive and haematogenous less so
*Uncommon*
2. Minimal change nephrotic syndrome
*Rare*
3. Congenital disorders: cystinosis, renal tubular acidosis

### Childhood
*Common*
1. Overt urinary tract infection and 'asymptomatic' bacteriuria (females >males, ratio 50:1)
*Uncommon*
2. Acute and chronic glomerulonephritis

## COMMON FINDINGS

### Boys
1. Prepuce: retractile by 3 years in most boys, but, providing the opening is not scarred and there is no ballooning of the foreskin on micturition, not to be retractile is normal even in late childhood
2. Testes: in scrotum by 1 year, unless:
    (i) Absent bilaterally: consider intersex problems
    (ii) Maldescended: after emerging from the superficial inguinal ring the testis goes ectopic, to the superficial inguinal pouch, femoral, perineal or pubic area. Torsion may occur
    (iii) Undescended: normal line of descent, but arrested intra-abdominally, in the inguinal canal or high in the neck of the scrotum. Hernia common, fertility poor, malignancy more likely than in maldescent
    (iv) Retractile: caused by cold hands or anxiety and descend if the child squats. If this manoeuvre fails, see (i)–(iii) above
3. Hydrocoeles: commoner in premature boys, gone by 1 year, transilluminate, and fingers can get above them, unlike inguinal hernias

### Girls
1. Perineum and vaginal mucosa pink prepubertally, darkening to becoming velvety red in puberty
2. Slight clear or white vaginal discharge is normal

## CAUSES OF FREQUENT MICTURITION

1. Physiological: age related
2. Emotional: stress, attention seeking
3. Urinary tract: infection, gross reflux, obstructive uropathy (e.g. neurogenic bladder, posterior urethral valves causing dribbling, poor stream)
4. Diabetes mellitus

## CAUSES OF POLYURIA

1. Psychological
2. Urinary tract infection
3. Diabetes mellitus and diabetes insipidus

## CAUSES OF ENURESIS

See p 27.

## CAUSES OF COLOURED URINE

1. Dark yellow: concentrated (may cause red 'spot' of urates on napkin in boys and can be mistaken for haematuria), bile
2. Pink to dark red: blood, food dyes, beeturia, dyes, drugs, e.g. senna

## CAUSES OF HAEMATURIA

(May be microscopic)

1. Trauma to kidneys, renal tract
2. Urinary tract infection
3. Acute glomerulonephritis
4. Henoch-Schönlein (anaphylactoid) purpura
5. Recurrent haematuria syndrome occurring with fevers and upper respiratory tract infections
6. Wilms' tumour (rare)

## CAUSES OF ACUTE RENAL FAILURE BY AGE AT PRESENTATION

| Prerenal (pump failure, loss of fluid) | Renal | Postrenal (obstructive) |
|---|---|---|
| Common | Uncommon | Rare |
| **Infants** | | |
| Acute D and V Septicaemia, congenital heart disease | UTI Haemolytic–uraemic syndrome* | Posterior urethral valves |
| **Children** | | |
| Dehydration, trauma (acute blood loss), burns, scalds (protein loss) | Acute glomerulonephritis Acute tubular necrosis from prerenal cause | Neurogenic, i.e. spinal cord abnormality/ damage |

*Haemolytic uraemic syndrome is uncommon, usually occurring in children under 1 year old, with infection, pallor, coma, fits; often hypertensive; may die. Laboratory findings: haemolytic anaemia, fragmented red cells, raised blood urea.
D and V = diarrhoea and vomiting; UTI = urinary tract infection.

## CAUSES OF CHRONIC RENAL FAILURE

1. Reflux nephropathy is commonest in UK — Late childhood
2. Haemolytic uraemic syndrome — Infancy onwards
3. Chronic glomerulonephritis — Late childhood
4. Renal hypoplasia or dysplasia and polycystic kidney disease — Early, often in infancy

## COMMON FEATURES OF ACUTE NEPHRITIS AND NEPHROTIC SYNDROME

|  | Nephritis | Nephrosis |
|---|---|---|
| Cause | Group Aβ *H. streptococcus*, Henoch-Schönlein, idiopathic | Unknown in 90% |
| Age (years) | 5–15, rarely preschool | Mainly preschool, up to 10 |
| Onset | Sudden | Days or weeks |
| Mode | Haematuria | Oedema |
| Temperature | Raised | Normal |
| BP | May be raised | Normal |
| Urine | | |
| protein | ++/+++ | ++++ (Albustix) |
| blood | ++/+++ | Absent |
| casts | Red cell | Hyaline/fatty |
| Plasma protein | Normal | Low albumin |
| Cholesterol | Normal | Raised |
| ASOT | Raised | Normal |
| C3 complement | Low | Normal |
| Prognosis | Good In 95% | Good unless raised blood urea/BP, haematuria, age <1 or >10 years |

## CAUSES OF RENAL MASSES

1. Unilateral cystic kidney, hydronephrosis, trauma, Wilms' tumour
2. Bilateral
   (i) Hydronephrosis from obstruction
   (ii) Cystic disease, infantile and adult forms
   (iii) Tumour, e.g. Wilms'

## RENAL TUBULAR ACIDOSIS (RTA)

RTA is commonly due to a loss of bicarbonate from the proximal tubules, causing a metabolic acidosis. The Fanconi syndrome comprises RTA, glycosuria, aminoaciduria and excessive loss of phosphate and electrolytes, which is due to renal tubular damage secondary to lead poisoning or inborn errors of metabolism or is idiopathic with no known cause.

# Metabolic disorders

## ACID–BASE DISORDERS

Infants have lower plasma concentrations of bicarbonate (18–24 mmol/l) than older children and adults, because the renal threshold is lower. They are therefore less able to acidify their urine and have less reserve (or defence) against acidosis.

### Characteristics of acid–base disorders

|  | pH | $pCO_2$ | Base excess | Standard bicarbonate ($HCO_3^-$) |
|---|---|---|---|---|
| Metabolic acidosis | Down | Down* | − n | Down |
| Metabolic alkalosis | Up | Up* | + n | Up |
| Respiratory acidosis | Down | Up | + n | Up* |
| Respiratory alkalosis | Up | Down | − n | Down* |

\* After allowing time for compensation: quick respiratory (minutes), slow metabolic (hours)
n = Number of mmol/l of acid (−) or alkali (+) to be corrected to achieve 'neutrality'
Correction of negative base excess (base deficit):
   body weight (kg) × base deficit × 0.3
   = number of mmol alkali (sodium bicarbonate) needed

## IMPORTANT CAUSES OF ACID–BASE DISORDERS

1. Metabolic acidosis (see Anion Gap below for further help in differentiation)
    (i) Loss of bicarbonate: diarrhoea, renal tubular acidosis
    (ii) Gain of strong acid: starvation, diabetes mellitus, shock, septicaemia, rarely renal failure and inborn errors of metabolism
2. Metabolic alkalosis: pyloric stenosis

3. Respiratory acidosis
    (i) Central: depressed brain stem, e.g. drugs, infection
    (ii) Obstructive: asthma, foreign body, epiglottitis
    (iii) Lung disease: respiratory distress syndrome (often a mixed respiratory and metabolic acidosis), cystic fibrosis
4. Respiratory alkalosis: hysteria, encephalitis, early salicylate poisoning, compensatory for metabolic acidosis

## ANION GAP

Estimating the anion gap is useful in differentiating causes of metabolic acidosis. As an approximation the anion gap = plasma $(Na^+ + K^+) - (Cl^- + HCO_3^-)$ and is normally 14–20 mmol/l
1. Normal anion gap, with hyperchloraemia
    (i) Loss of bicarbonate: diarrhoea, renal bicarbonate wasting
    (ii) Failure to regenerate bicarbonate: renal tubular acidosis
2. Increased anion gap
    (i) (a) Excessive production of lactic acid from:
            — work of breathing and/or hypoxia in asthma and respiratory distress syndrome (RDS)
            — septicaemia, underperfusion, shock
            — some rare metabolic errors, e.g. von Gierke's glycogen storage disorder: hypoglycaemia, enlarged kidneys and liver, FTT, learning disability; later xanthoma, gout
        (b) Keto acids: starvation, diabetes mellitus
    (ii) Reduced glomerular filtration rate and ingestion of milk which contains sulphated amino acids which metabolize to sulphuric acid. Excess protein or phosphate from cow's milk is significant in prematures and renal failure
    (iii) Ingestion of salicylates, ethylene glycol
    (iv) Inborn errors → amino acid ketones, e.g. maple syrup urine disease

## HYPOCALCAEMIA

Normal values by age:
Newborn    >1.8 mmol/l (may be lower in premature infants)
Older      >2.1 mmol/l

### Causes

*Common*
1. Newborn: stress, cow's milk, maternal vitamin D deficiency
2. Hyperventilation due to stress, in older children and adolescents
*Uncommon* (unless nutritionally disposed, e.g. Asian diet and low vitamin D intake)

3. Rickets
*Rare*
4. Renal rickets
5. Endocrine: Addison's disease, hypoparathyroidism

## CAUSES OF HYPOGLYCAEMIA

NB: Neonatal hypoglycaemia see p14.
A. Ketotic
*Common*
1. Malnutrition
2. Stress, e.g. septicaemia, hypothermia
*Uncommon*
3. Fasting (previously called ketotic hypoglycaemia): usually 1–3
   years old, thin, low birth weight
4. Alcohol (particularly likely after ingestion in children)
*Rare but important*
5. Reye's syndrome of hepatic failure, cerebral oedema with
   acidosis and hypoglycaemia after viral infection, may be
   exacerbated by salicylates
6. Hypopituitarism
B. Non-ketotic
7. Hyperinsulinism, usually a diabetic child, but beware
   'Munchausen by proxy'

## INBORN ERRORS OF METABOLISM

Single enzyme deficiency, usually inherited as autosomal recessive
(p 2), occasionally sex linked.

## AMINOACIDURIA

Increased levels in both blood and urine in inborn error, e.g.
phenylketonuria, or urine alone in renal tubular damage (p 79).

### Phenylketonuria
Deficiency of phenylalanine hydroxylase results in fair haired, blue
eyed, eczematous children with mental retardation and fits.
'Mousey' smell. Guthrie test screens for raised phenylalanine blood
level.
   Treatment: Diet low in phenylalanine, e.g. 'lofenalac' milk.

### Maple syrup urine disease
Deficiency of a branched chain decarboxylase causes high levels of
leucine, isoleucine and valine, and urine smells like maple syrup
(caramel). Within days or weeks of birth, vomiting, severe
metabolic acidosis, seizures, hypoglycaemia, coma and death
unless special diet given.

# Orthopaedics

## NORMAL POSTURAL VARIATIONS

Neonate: Intrauterine position commonly causes postural deformities of feet.
Infant: Pigeon toe (metatarsus varus) is normal if passively correctable. Curly, overlapping toes usually self correct.
Toddler: Flat feet and bow legs to 2 years.
Preschool: Knock-knees, mild. More severe suggests rickets.

**Note**
1. Asymmetry is always suspicious: consider congenital abnormality, trauma or tumour
2. Symmetrical deformity: endocrine or metabolic disorder is more likely

## CAUSES OF SCOLIOSIS

1. Primary: postural, and infantile and adolescent types
2. Secondary
    (i) Bone: hemivertebrae
    (ii) Neurogenic: spina bifida, poliomyelitis, cerebral palsy
    (iii) Ligaments: Marfan's syndrome of tall stature, wide arm span, long digits, lens dislocation, aortic rupture, scoliosis. Autosomal dominant inheritance
    (iv) Muscle: muscular dystrophies

## CAUSES OF ACUTE PAINFUL JOINT OR LIMP

Remember, 'growing pains' and cramps are two common conditions with characteristic histories which must be differentiated from the following causes:
1. Trauma
    (i) Severe
    (ii) Mild, may exacerbate slipped femoral epiphysis (see p 85)
    (iii) Non-accidental injury
2. Irritable hip
3. Infection: osteomyelitis especially *S. aureus, H. influenzae*, TB, viral, e.g. mumps, rubella
4. Henoch-Schönlein purpura (p 54)
5. Osteochondritis, e.g. Perthe's disease of the hip
6. Haematological: sickle cell disease, leukaemia
7. Rheumatic fever
8. Iatrogenic: drug reaction, serum sickness

## CAUSES OF CHRONIC ARTHRITIS

1. Infective: mycoplasma pneumoniae, brucellosis, TB
2. Postinfective: salmonella, shigella
3. Juvenile rheumatoid arthritis (JRA) or Still's disease
4. Chronic bowel disease: Crohn's, ulcerative colitis

## CAUSES OF ARTHRITIS BY DIFFERENTIATION OF ACUTE/CHRONIC, AFEBRILE/TEMPERATURE

| Onset | Afebrile | Febrile |
|---|---|---|
| Acute | Trauma, haemorrhage, tumour Fracture through bone cyst | Septic arthritis/osteomyelitis Irritable hip (low grade fever) |
| Chronic | Asymmetrical leg length, Perthe's CNS: cerebral palsy, polio, myopathy | Juvenile chronic arthritis, TB |

## DIFFERENTIAL DIAGNOSIS OF STILL'S DISEASE, RHEUMATIC FEVER AND HENOCH-SCHÖNLEIN (ANAPHYLACTOID) PURPURA

See p 54.

## DIFFERENTIAL DIAGNOSIS OF PATHOLOGY IN HIP, WITH PAIN IN HIP OR REFERRED TO KNEE

(Painful legs are generally held in the position of comfort, abducted, flexed and externally rotated)

| | Age (years) | Clinical, duration of symptoms | Investigations |
|---|---|---|---|
| 'Irritable hip' | 3–10 | Usually boy, well, limping, slight temperature Hours to days | Normal FBC, ESR |
| Septic hip | 0–5+ | Toxic, any movement painful +++ Hours to 1–2 days | Blood culture normal at first, WBC++; aspirate early |
| TB | 2–15 | Subacute, stiff and very painful. Psoas abcess common Weeks to months | CXR: Hilar glands? Do Hb and WBC, ESR, Mantoux, urine for AAFB |
| Perthe's | 5–10 | Usually boy, well, bilateral occasionally May take months for diagnosis, 2–4 years to resolve | X-ray: widened joint space → denser femoral head → fragmentation |
| Juvenile chronic arthritis | 1–15 | Pain, morning stiffness. Systemic disease + rash in 'Still's disease' type Minimum 6–12 weeks for diagnosis | Raised ESR, raised anti-nuclear antibodies in pauciarticular |
| Slipped femoral epiphysis | 10–15 | Fat tall boys >girls, well, hip flexion → external rotation. Bilateral in 20% Acute: minutes. Subacute/chronic days to weeks | X-ray: capital epiphysis falling back and downward in lateral view |

AAFB = acid and alcohol fast bacilli (tuberculosis)

# Dermatology

## COMMON SKIN CONDITIONS CAUSING DIAGNOSTIC CONFUSION

### Napkin dermatitis, intertrigo, seborrhoeic eczema and atopic eczema

| Age (months) | Cause | Clinical | Prognosis |
|---|---|---|---|
| 1–6 | **Napkin dermatitis** Prolonged skin contact with urine soaked nappy. Worse with faeces, may even cause ammonia burns | Groin folds spared, red, scald like or ulcers ('burns'), often infected | Good |
| 0.5–12 | **Intertrigo** Friction between folds of skin plus water/sweat | Fat babies, neck, axilla, groin; candida 'satellite' lesions common | Good |
| 0.5–3 | **Seborrhoea** Excess sebum production from sweat glands | Non-itchy, red skin and yellow greasy scales Spread: scalp, behind ears, neck, axillae; napkin area affected up to 8 months old | Good |
| 3–24 | **Atopic eczema** Inherited | Itchy ++ Spread: scalp, face to extensor surfaces of the limbs; later to flexures. Strep. and Staph. infections occur readily, occasionally H. simplex | Depends on age at onset: Under 2 years old is good, older is poorer |

## Erythema

*Erythema nodosum*
Raised red nodules over shins, rarely thighs, forearms
Causes
1. Unknown
2. Infections: group A β-haemolytic streptococcus (βHS), viruses, TB
3. Drugs, e.g. penicillin, sulphonamides

*Erythema multiforme*
Wheals, red/purple target lesions, ulcers at mucocutaneous junctions. If severe called Stevens-Johnson syndrome
Causes
1. Unknown
2. Infection, e.g. *H. simplex, M. pneumoniae*
3. Drugs, e.g. phenobarbitone

*Toxic erythema*
Scarlet fever or measles like rash, followed by generalized peeling of skin
Causes
1. β-haemolytic streptococcus
2. Drugs
3. Unknown
(Differential diagnosis includes Kawasaki disease, characterized by conjunctival injection, ulcers to oropharynx, swelling of hands and feet, lymphadenopathy and cardiac involvement)

## DIFFERENTIAL DIAGNOSIS OF HENOCH-SCHÖNLEIN PURPURA (ANAPHYLACTOID) FROM IDIOPATHIC THROMBOCYTOPENIA (ITP)

| Age (years) | Cause | Clinical | Prognosis | Investigations |
|---|---|---|---|---|
| **Henoch-Schönlein** | | | | |
| 2–7 | β Haem. strep. Foods? Viral Unknown | 1. Oedema, erythema, purpura over extensor surfaces 2. Small joints swell 3. Colicky abdomen 4. Haematuria | Recurs for 7–10 weeks, for up to 2 years | Normal coagulation, normal capillary resistance |
| **ITP** | | | | |
| Any | Immune, occasionally rubella | Sudden onset, well, generalized purpura; bleeding from mouth and nose, and haematuria, especially likely if becomes chronic | Good in 90%. Remainder 10% persist for >6 months, labelled chronic | Platelets low, bleeding time prolonged |

# Management of common problems and emergencies

## AIRWAY/RESPIRATORY EMERGENCIES

### Acute epiglottitis
Symptoms of stridor, drooling, fever in a 3–7 year old who becomes toxic within a few hours, due to *H. influenzae* b (Hib) found in throat and blood cultures. *Do not try to visualize the epiglottis* as this may precipitate a respiratory arrest. Introduction of Hib vaccination has caused great reduction in incidence.

*Management*
1. Move to nearest intensive treatment unit (ITU), meanwhile nebulize adrenaline 1 in 10000 to reduce swelling
2. Endotracheal intubation for 1–2 days likely to be needed
3. Humidified air/oxygen
4. Cefotaxime I.v. preferred to chloramphenicol/ampicillin because of possible Hib antibiotic resistance

NB: Remember foreign body (FB) commonly, retropharyngeal abscess occasionally, diphtheria rarely may present in a similar way. See p 44 for comparison of FB, epiglottitis and laryngotracheo bronchitis.

### Acute croup
Inspiratory stridor usually preceded by a few days' 'cold', though this is not always so and can easily appear like an epiglottitis. Age is 6 months to 3 years old, mild fever and constitutional upset. Wheeze common.

*Management*
Humidify air/oxygen, no antibiotic. Rarely is intubation necessary.

### Acute respiratory failure
*Causes*
1. Central: head injury, drugs, convulsion, infection
2. Airway: acute epiglottitis, foreign body
3. Parenchymal: pneumonia, bronchiolitis, asthma
4. Chest wall: polio, trauma

*Clinical*
Restless, agitated from hypoxia, cyanosis, silent chest not moving sufficient air.
   Blood gases: Low $PaO_2$ in oxygen (<8 kPa (55 mmHg) in 40% oxygen) and/or rising $CO_2$ in oxygen (>8 kPa in 80% oxygen).

*Management*
Secure airway, initially ventilate by bag and mask, proceed to intubate, assist ventilation. Deal with primary cause.

**Acute bronchiolitis**
'Cold' is followed, 3–5 days later, by progressive cough, wheeze, difficulty in feeding, signs as for asthma (below), often fine inspiratory crepitations, in infant 6 weeks to 6 months old; due to respiratory syncitial virus (RSV).

*Management*
1. Oxygen
2. Suction of secretions
3. Tube feeding or i.v. fluids if unable to feed orally
4. Antibiotics rarely indicated. Ribovirin for infants with bronchopulmonary dysplasia or CHD is of doubtful efficacy
5. Bronchodilators: Ipratropium bromide (Atrovent) nebulizers may be effective in 40%. Generally unresponsive to β-agonists

May recur. Most grow out of their wheezy episodes by 2 years old. Only a third later develop asthma.

**Acute asthma**
From 1 year old, expiratory wheeze, difficulty in speaking, head extended, nostrils flared, chest increased anteroposterior diameter, accessory muscles working, rapid pulse, may have pulsus paradoxus (pulse weaker on inspiration), cyanosis in air.
   Precipitants: URTI, exercise, changes in weather, emotional, aero-allergens (pollens, house dust mite, animals) and food allergens.

*Status asthmaticus: indications for hospitalization*
1. Cyanosis
2. Drowsy/semicomatose
3. Unable to speak or feed
4. PEFR <50% of expected after a $β_2$-bronchodilator
5. Failure to respond to inhaled $β_2$-bronchodilator and/or as bad within 1 hour of its use
6. Previous severe attack, e.g. collapse/ventilated

*Management of acute episode: stepwise approach*

Step 1   Nebulized sympathomimetic, e.g. salbutamol, to be
         repeated according to response
         Ipratropium may be added if severe attack
         Oxygen immediately if hypoxic/cyanosed. If on inhaled
         steroid, double dose until asymptomatic for 7 days
Step 2   Oral prednisolone 2 mg/kg for 3 days if previously given
         steroids or more than a single dose of nebulized drug
         required
Step 3   Consider continuous infusion of i.v. fluid and
         hydrocortisone and theophylline i.v., avoiding loading
         dose if already on oral treatment or $\beta_2$-agonist
         (salbutamol/terbutaline) i.v. bolus followed by continuous
         infusion

NB. Antibiotics only if good evidence of infection. Monitor pulse,
respiration; chest X-ray and blood gases in severe or deteriorating
episode.

## Chronic asthma
*Diagnosis*
1. Repeated episodes of cough, dyspnoea and wheeze; ± presence
   of infantile eczema and atopic family history
2. A reduction of 15–20% in PEFR in an exercise test, or increase
   of >15% in PEFR following $\beta_2$-agonist inhalation
3. Clinical response to a trial of a bronchodilating drug

*Management:*
A partnership between the patient, the family and the health
professionals

Needs:
   (i) Understanding the condition
   (ii) Monitoring of symptoms, peak flow and drug usage
   (iii) Prearranged action plan
   (iv) Written guidelines
1. Patient/parent education. Assessment of severity. Match drug
   delivery system to child's ability to use it with benefit. Frequent
   checks on inhaler techniques; check compliance. The aim is to
   facilitate a normal life
2. Sporting performance impaired by exercise-induced
   bronchoconstriction can be helped by pre-activity inhaled
   $\beta_2$-agonist or cromoglycate 5 minutes before
3. Environmental factors:
   (i) Stop smoking
   (ii) Avoid allergens if realistic
4. Learning and emotional problems: school non-attendance and
   learning difficulties resulting; within the family, discussion,
   psychotherapy

5. Home monitoring: the Daily Record Card
   (i) PEFR below 80% of predicted is abnormal. Start/intensify treatment
   (ii) Below 60% significant airway obstruction. Intensify treatment, as agreed or consult with doctor
   (iii) Below 25% is an emergency, requiring urgent medical advice in hospital

**Treatment algorithm for chronic asthma**

Mild        Inhaled $\beta_2$-agonist intermittently
                  ↓
                  >3 doses per week
                  ↓
Moderate  Add cromoglycate (CGC), or low-dose inhaled steroids# if inadequate response to CGC in 6 weeks
                  ↓
Severe     Consider   1. Long acting $\beta_2$-agonists
                      2. Slow release theophylline
                      3. Ipratropium bromide
                  ↓
Very severe  Increase inhaled steroids, consider oral steroids

#Inhaled steroids up to 400 μg daily. If controlled decrease dose after 3 months. If uncontrolled, increase to 600 μg daily.

**Pneumonia**
Bronchopneumonia commoner then lobar pneumonia, especially in the preschool child.

*Causes*
Primary viral or bacterial, or secondary, e.g. post measles, whooping cough, milk inhalation, an underlying abnormality, e.g. cystic fibrosis.

*Clinical*
Babies may be very ill, grey, cyanosed, respiratory rate and effort increased, and the episode complicated by a febrile convulsion.
    In older children lobar pneumonia can mimic acute appendicitis, and meningism may suggest meningitis. Upper respiratory 'rattle' due to pharyngeal secretions not to be confused with fine crackles from parenchymal fluid, or the coarse crackles from fluid/secretions in bronchi.

*Investigations*
Chest X-ray, Hb and WBC, throat swab, blood culture, Mantoux, according to severity. If episodes recur consider sweat test (after the first if staphylococcus/pseudomonas), look for foreign body or immune deficiency.

*Management*
Suck out secretions from the airway, give physiotherapy, oxygen and nasogastric or i.v. feeds according to need. Antibiotics in clinical favour include cefotaxime, ampicillin, or gentamicin and penicillin in sick infants. Erythromycin is preferred for most community acquired infections, mycoplasma pneumonia or penicillin allergy.

## CARDIAC EMERGENCIES

### Cardiac failure
*Symptoms to note*
Lethargy, feeding problems or breathless on feeding, sweating, failure to thrive, recent excessive weight gain or oedema, blue attacks. Often seems precipitated or exacerbated by an intercurrent illness, e.g. pneumonia.

*Signs*
Rapid pulse and respiration, hepatomegaly, wheeze, excessive weight gain. Check femoral pulses and BP, heart sounds, murmurs (p 47).

*Investigations*
Chest X-ray, ECG, Hb, WBC, E and U, blood gases, glucose, bacteriology.

*Management*
1. Prop up, give oxygen 30%, nasogastric feeds in infants
2. Correct biochemical abnormalities: acidosis, hypoglycaemia, hypocalcaemia
3. Sedation if restless: phenobarbitone preferred to opiates
4. Diuretic, e.g. frusemide, consider potassium supplements unless spironolactone added
5. Vasodilator to reduce after-load, e.g. Captopril. Now preferred to digoxin especially in high output states, e.g. VSD
6. Treat precipitating event, i.e. anaemia or infection. Monitor weight, pulse, respirations, liver size

### Cardiorespiratory arrest
Remember 'A-B-C-D-E'

*Airway*
Clear mucus/vomit with swab round finger/suction. (Meconium in newborn should be aspirated as head is delivered; if fresh, intubate and apply suction with wide bore catheter or suction direct to the end of endotracheal tube.)

*Breathing*
Baby's nose and mouth covered in mouth to mouth, older children mouth only. Give a breath according to size, ensuring the chest moves with each breath. Bag and mask: use plastic airway, be sure mask seal on face is tight, support jaw.

*Cardiac output*
Failure of pump or blood volume
| | |
|---|---|
| Pump: | 1. Neonate, use 2 fingers on mid-sternum |
| | 2. <1 year old, circle chest with hands, thumbs pressing down on mid-sternum |
| | 3. >1 year old, use heel of hand on mid to lower sternum |
| Rate: | 1 breath to 5 compressions at 80–100 compressions per minute |
| Effectiveness: | Carotid/femoral pulse felt |
| Blood volume: | Plasma expander or 0.9% saline 20 ml/kg in hypovolaemic shock |

*Drugs*
| | |
|---|---|
| A-B-C-D: | Adrenaline/atropine/antidote (e.g. naloxone in the newborn) |
| | Bicarbonate |
| | Calcium salts |
| | Dextrose |

*Electrocardiograph*
Electrocardiograph for arrhythmias.
   NB: Continue attempts beyond half an hour even if no heart beat if hypothermia from cold water immersion, or drug ingestion suspected.


## BURNS AND SCALDS

### Immediate action in the home
1. Scald: strip off affected clothing, as it retains the hot liquid
2. Scald/burn: if small immerse in cold running water, or add ice to a basin of cold water, until cool. Cover area in a clean dry sheet, towel or dressing

### Hospital assessment
1. Airway (respiratory tract burn likely if soot in nostrils, or wheezy)
2. Appropriate analgesia, e.g. morphine i.v.
3. Plasma expanders if >10% of surface affected, to prevent shock, renal failure. Colloid (plasma/plasma protein fraction/Haemaccel) or Ringer's solution. Blood in full thickness (FT) burn/scald
4. Weigh

5. Hb check for early haemoconcentration, and subsequent anaemia in full thickness burn
6. Monitor urine output, blood and urine biochemistry, beware of renal failure

NB: Rule of 9s does not apply, e.g. infant head 18%, legs 13%, arms 9%, trunk 18% front/back.
   Remember full thickness is anaesthetic to pin prick.
   Consider non-accidental injury, especially in a preschool child.

## OTHER ACUTE INFECTIONS

### Acute diarrhoea
Diarrhoea constitutes an increase in frequency and fluid content of stools.

*Clinical signs*
Clinical signs of isotonic dehydration as a percentage loss of body weight:
5% (mild − 50 ml/kg): lethargic, loss of skin turgor, dry mouth, fontanelle slack
10% (moderate = 100 ml/kg): also tachycardia, tachypnoea, fontanelle and eyes sunken, mottled skin, oliguria
15% (severe = 150 ml/kg): also shock, coma, hypotension
   Symptoms occur earlier in hypotonic dehydration (serum sodium <130 mmol/l), later in hypernatraemic (>150 mmol/l) dehydration.

*Investigations*
In all but mild cases, do Hb, WBC, E and U, bacteriology of stool (×3), throat, urine and blood
1. Route of administration and initial resuscitation
   Oral or nasogastric feeds unless unconscious, absent bowel sounds, 10% or more dehydrated or shocked. In shock give plasma or 0.9% saline i.v. 20 ml/kg over 20 minutes. If i.v. fluids are needed give 4% dextrose/0.18% saline for 24 hours. Bicarbonate may be given if acidosis is severe, but care is needed (see diabetic ketoacidosis)
2. R+M+O
   Replacement = percentage dehydration (above)
   Maintenance (up to 10 kg = 100 ml/kg/day, next 10–25 kg = add 50 ml/kg/day, >25 kg add 25 ml/kg/day)
   Ongoing losses from vomiting or diarrhoea
3. Oral rehydration solution (ORS)
   Recommended by the World Health Organization (WHO) for developing countries; contains sodium 90 mmol/l, potassium 30 mmol/l, bicarbonate 30 mmol/l, chloride 90 mmol/l and glucose

2% (110 mmol/l). Developed countries still prefer an ORS with lower sodium (30–50 mmol/l) and often a higher sugar content (4%), e.g. Diorylate

4. Method
Administer ORS little and often (5–10 ml every 1–5 minutes is WHO policy) to replace deficit in 6 hours, offering extra after each vomit or diarrhoea. Breast feeding should continue. Water may be offered after the diarrhoea has eased, or in a ratio of 2 ORS: 1 water during rehydration

5. Reintroduce whole/powdered undiluted cow's milk within a day, starches (potato, rice) within 1–2 days. Soy milk may be preferred for a few days to avoid the usually transient post enteritis lactose/cow's milk intolerance

6. Hypernatraemic dehydration
The deficit is corrected more slowly, over 24–72 hours to avoid convulsions.
Monitor urine output for signs of renal failure, weigh regularly, investigate blood biochemistry and gases as required

## Meningitis, acute bacterial

Initial signs may be non-specific in the infant, e.g. initially presenting as gastroenteritis. Irritable cry, coma, convulsion, apnoea, signs of a bulging fontanelle, head retraction and resistance to flexion. (Meningism is a feature of respiratory infections, but lumbar puncture (LP) must be considered.)

Associated conditions are common, e.g. otitis media and purpura in meningococcal infection. Onset is rapid in the neonate, and in pneumococcal or meningococcal infection, and is often preceded by a 'cold' for some days before if *H. influenzae.*

*Investigations*
CSF cells, Gram stain and glucose, bacteriology, Hb, WBC, E and U, blood glucose, chest X-ray

*Diagnosis*
CSF turbid, polymorphs >20/mm$^3$, protein >0.45 g/l, glucose <2/3 blood glucose

*Treatment*
Initialy, until culture and sensitivities are known:
Neonate: *E. coli*, group $\beta$ haemolytic streptococcus likely, listeria possible therefore a newer cephalosporin and/or gentamycin is given with amoxycillin. Treat for 3 weeks.
After 3 months old: *H. influenzae*, meningococcus and pneumococcus likely, therefore cefotaxime is preferred to ampicillin in high dose, plus chloramphenicol in case *H. influenzae* is resistant. Treat for 10 days.

*Important complications*
1. Convulsions
2. Cerebral oedema, subdural effusion, hydrocephalus
3. Hyponatraemia from inappropriate antidiuretic hormone release
4. Deafness: always screen hearing immediately on recovery
5. Drug fever: rise of fever after initial fall
6. Long term: mental handicap, cerebral palsy, epilepsy, deaf

**Osteomyelitis/septic arthritis**
Reluctance to use a limb, local swelling or tenderness may progress to a 'toxic' looking septicaemic infant or child (50% <2 years old). History of injury in a third. Usually a single joint, hip >knee >ankle >elbow, metaphyseal spread via blood stream in 90%, direct in 10%; often to the joint in infancy as vessels pass through the growth plate into the epiphysis. Direct spread to the hip is frequent as the femoral metaphysis lies in the joint space; early diagnosis and treatment are vital in preventing damage to the femoral head.

*Investigations*
Blood culture, Hb, WBC, X-rays. Aspiration of bone/joint

*Treatment*
Intravenous antibiotics, in expectation of a penicillinase producing *Staphylococcus aureus* (70% of cases). Flucloxacillin + fucidin + ampicillin/cefuroxime is a popular combination. Immobilize the limb, watch.
Surgery is indicated immediately in septic hip in infants and, if poor response to treatment after 24 hours, in older children.

**Urinary tract infection**
*Clinical*
1. Neonate: poor feeding, vomiting, fever, weight loss, conjugated jaundice, boys >girls
2. Preschool: vomiting, diarrhoea, failure to thrive, irritability and crying, fever, girls:boys = 50:1 from now on
3. School age: localization of pain to suprapubic or loin area, fever, polydipsia, polyuria, dysuria

NB: Dysuria is also a symptom of vulvitis or balanitis in the older child and as likely as UTI if otherwise asymptomatic, but this is diagnosed only after appropriate investigation as the consequence of untreated UTI may be renal scarring.

*Investigations*
1. Check
    (i) Dip stick for nitrite and leucocyte esterase. These are
        unlikely to be negative if UTI is present
    (ii) Blood pressure, Hb, WBC, E and U, serum creatinine,
        urine ± blood culture (septicaemic?)
2. Imaging in *all* cases, according to age:
    (i) Immediate: ultrasound (US) to look for calyceal dilatation
        from infection or obstruction of ureters; plain X-ray for
        stones, spinal anomalies
    (ii) Urgent if US in boy shows bilateral dilated upper renal tract:
        micturating cystourethrogram (MCUG) for posterior urethral
        valves
    (iii) After 4–8 weeks: kidney X-ray and radioisotope studies for
        scarring, pelvi-ureteric obstruction and ureteral reflux,
        duplex collecting systems, bladder diverticuli

Imaging investigations by age at presentation and number of
infections suffered

| <1 year old | 1–5 years old | >5 years old |
| --- | --- | --- |
| US, DMSA, MCUG in *all* cases | 1. *First infection:* US, plain X-ray abdomen, DMSA (IVP if DMSA unavailable) <br> 2. *Second infection or scar found.* MCG for VUR | 1. US, plain X-ray abdomen <br> 2. DMSA and DTPA *only* if scarring is found |

DMSA = dimercaptosuccinic acid; DTPA = diethylenetriamine pentacetic
    acid; MCG = micturating cystogram; VUR = vesicoureteric reflux.

*Bacteriology*
<1 year old = *E. coli*
>1 year old = 1/3 each *E. coli*, proteus, others

Significance of colony counts in the diagnosis of UTI:
1. $10^5$/ml or more in a clean catch (CCU) or midstream urine
    (MSU), in at least 2 separate samples
2. $10^4$/ml via catheter
3. Any growth on suprapubic urine (SPU) obtained by bladder
    puncture
4. Only *no* growth in a single bag urine (contamination is so likely,
    do CCU/MSU/SPU for confirmatory proof of infection)
Pus cells in urine: may be *absent* in urinary infection, yet up to
$100/mm^3$ in girl's bag urine, or more if vulvitis, or in a boy with
balanitis.

Treat according to antibiotic sensitivities; give i.v. gentamycin + ampicillin if septicaemic, fluids ++. Prophylaxis with trimethoprim 2 mg/kg at night until renal investigations complete for children under 2 years old.

## MISCELLANEOUS PROBLEMS

### Diabetic ketoacidosis
Polydipsia, polyuria for days or weeks only. Weight loss, dehydration, vomiting, abdominal pain ('appendicitis?'), deep breaths ('pneumonia', 'uraemia'?), infection associated, e.g. urinary infection or 'thrush', coma ('hypoglycaemia'?). Check weight, assess dehydration

*Investigations*
Blood glucose, blood gases, E and U, Hb and WBC, bacteriology.

*Management*

*Severe ketoacidosis*
1. Rehydrate using 0.9% saline. Requirement = per cent dehydration (10% = 100 ml/kg) plus maintenance (50–100 ml/kg) intravenously, adding potassium as urine flow recommences and as serum biochemistry indicates
2. Insulin, soluble. Initial bolus 0.1–0.5 U/kg, then i.v. infusion or hourly i.m. injections (0.1 U/kg/hour) until blood glucose falls to 15 mmol/l, when 4% glucose/0.18% saline infusion replaces 0.9% saline, and soluble insulin is then given every 4–6 hours
3. Bicarbonate is now rarely given because $HCO_3 \rightleftharpoons HO^- + CO_2$, and $CO_2$ crosses into the brain, where $CO_2 + H_2O \rightleftharpoons H_2CO_3$, i.e. acid rises in the brain, delaying recovery of consciousness. Monitor input, output and biochemistry carefully

*Mild to moderate ketoacidosis, or in recovery phase from severe*
1. Insulin, soluble 0.5 U/kg subcutaneously before each main meal, until blood glucose <15 mmol/l and no more ketonuria. Urine tests for glucose can be used in a sliding scale. Now consider long term insulin. Soluble twice daily in 0–3 year olds, 1 or 2 injections of medium acting insulin in middle childhood, and 2 of soluble plus medium acting insulin in adolescence. Inject before breakfast and main evening meal. Some teenagers will tolerate 4-injection regimens (soluble pre-meals, intermediate overnight)
2. Diet. Total calories = 1000 plus 100 per year of life, half as carbohydrate in 10g 'exchanges' for main meals and snacks between to avoid hypoglycaemia. Avoid extra fat, keeping it to one third of calories. High fibre foods are currently encouraged for their slower release of carbohydrates and hence less wide and wild excursions of blood glucose than with refined foods

**Hypoglycaemia**

*Definition*
This is related to age (see p14, 82).

*Signs*
The usual signs of hypoglycaemia are similar to those in adults.
The young child, however, may become drowsy or merely seem
more difficult than usual! The presence of ketones on the breath or
urine without hyperglycaemia/glycosuria is a sign of fasting
hypoglycaemia (ketotic hypoglycaemia), to which some small for
age preschool children are prone (p82).
  Beware of hypoglycaemia after ethyl alcohol ingestion in
children.

*Investigation*
Blood glucose, and insulin level if persistently low blood glucose
despite adequate treatment. Inappropriately high insulin for the low
blood glucose indicates hyperinsulinism (excess production by
pancreas/non-accidental administration). Low/normal c-peptide
level with high insulin level is diagnostic of exogenous insulin,
beware Munchausen by proxy!

*Management*
Oral glucose if able, otherwise i.v. glucose 0.5 g/kg body weight as
50% solution.

**Learning disorder/mental handicap**
An approach to diagnosis and management (also see Causes)

*Timing of presentation*
1. At birth (infection, drugs, alcohol, etc. in preganacy; appearance,
   e.g. Down's)
2. Parental suspicions
3. Detected at follow-up of difficult delivery, prematurity, or a
   severe illness, e.g. meningitis, prolonged seizure

*Pointers to mental handicap from the history*
1. Abnormal behaviour: excessively 'good', has to be woken for
   feeds, unresponsive, suspected of deafness
2. Abnormal motor patterns: floppy/stiff, preservation of primitive
   reflexes, later hyperactivity and repetitive stereotyped
   behaviour, e.g. turning on taps, rocking, running in circles
3. Failure to thrive, feeding difficulties
4. Delayed milestones of development

*Presence of an unusual marker to help 'spot' a syndrome*
1. Facial, e.g. Down's
2. Microcephaly and short stature, e.g. Seckel's bird headed dwarf

*Pitfalls (differential diagnosis)*
1. Normal variation, familial patterns of development
2. Lack of stimulation: inexperience, ignorance, deprivation, parental depression, abuse
3. Sensory disorder: deaf, partially sighted
4. Medical disease: malabsorption, acute illness
5. Autism
6. Degenerative disease, i.e. initially *normal* development

*Investigation*
1. For genetic disease: Wood's light for skin manifestations of tuberous sclerosis (TS), blood for hypercalcaemia, amino acids, thyroid function, urine for organic acids, mucopolysaccharides; if indicated, serology for TORCH, urine for cytomegalovirus
2. Chromosomes for suggestive signs, and fragile X examination in physically normal but learning disabled boys, especially with a family history, or if the mother is intellectually 'slow'
3. Skull X-ray for calcification due to TS and congenital infection. CT scan for suspected TS or structural abnormality, e.g. with cerebral palsy, seizures
4. EEG only if seizures are present

*Management*
1. Counselling and support of parents and siblings from the District Handicap Team.
Aims are:
   (a) To help come to terms with handicap
   (b) Enlist active participation in therapy
   (c) Anticipatory guidance to prevent or minimize difficult behaviour
Identification of a syndrome, e.g. Down's, fragile X, Prader-Willi, enables more accurate prediction of associated problems, levels of functioning, and prognosis, and reduces parental uncertainty
2. Assessment, needs, therapeutic programmes for stimulation (e.g. Portage scheme), speech, physiotherapy, self-help skills (see CP)
3. Notify Education Authority for instigation of a Statement of Special Needs
4. Behaviour modification for behaviour difficulties, e.g. head banging, self-mutilation, masturbation in public
5. Medication: for seizures, and overactivity if destructive and unmanageable

*Prognosis*
1. Life expectancy is reduced for ESN(S), especially in early childhood, due to respiratory infection, seizures, and associated congenital anomalies, e.g. cyanotic congenital heart disease in Down's
2. Psychological problems in 50% of ESN(S). 30% of ESN(M) also have behavioural and emotional difficulties
3. Majority of ESN(M) can be independent, in sheltered workshops, 'niche' employment, often living in sheltered accomodation. ESN(S) require constant supervision, with the family, or in a residential home or hostel sooner or later

*Prevention*
1. Antenatal diagnosis: for mothers >35 years old (Down's), inborn error of metabolism, or heritable brain malformation likely to show on US
2. Education about dangers of alcohol abuse
3. Universal immunization against rubella

**Poisoning**
*Immediate action in the home*
EXCEPT with volatile hydrocarbons or caustics or when child is unconscious, induce vomiting with fingers, *not* salt water, etc.

*Hospital assessment*
1. Establish a poison(s) has been taken, its name, amount, when, how. Consider non-accidental ingestion. Check with a National Poisons Information Service centre
2. Induce vomiting with syrup of ipecac, 15 ml + glass of water, within 6 hours of ingestion, up to 24 hours for salicylates. Repeat after 20 minutes if no result. Contraindicated in caustic, petrol or white spirit ingestion. Gastric lavage for the unconscious, with protected airway
3. Specific antidotes
   Acetyl cysteine/methionine, for paracetamol poisoning
   Activated charcoal for tricyclics, opiates or slow release theophylline poisoning
   Alkali diuresis for salicylate or phenobarbitone poisoning
   Desferrioxamine for iron
   Fuller's Earth for paraquat
   Glucose for alcohol (hypoglycaemia may be severe)
   Naloxone for Lomotil, opiates
   Oxygen for carbon monoxide poisoning, consider hyperbaric chamber
4. General measures: observation and, where appropriate, close monitoring of airway, circulation, temperature, fluid balance, blood glucose

## Pyrexia
A frequent presentation at all ages; most episodes are due to viral infection. Absence of localizing signs, at least initially, is common. Always consider contacts, foreign travel even up to a year ago (e.g. malaria), environmental hazards (pets, untreated milk, etc.).

Investigations in the acutely ill: bacterial 'screen', i.e. throat swab, stool, blood culture, urine. Lumbar puncture may be necessary. Hb, WBC, chest X-ray and Mantoux (thick film for malaria, serology for typhoid, hepatitis, glandular fever, etc., in appropriate cases). The ESR is often high in acute viral or bacterial infections, e.g. more chronic illness, TB, subacute bacterial endocarditis, collagenoses, malignancy, etc. In practice an 'infection screen' and blood culture, Hb, WBC and ESR, chest X-ray and Mantoux are done, followed by a period of observation. Only then are further tests likely to be helpful. Always consider Kawasaki's (p 54)

## Seizures
The most common cause is a febrile convulsion. In the absence of fever, epilepsy must be considered. Status epilepticus is a fit lasting more than 30 minutes or several fits with failure to regain consciousness between them.

## Action
1. Move child away from danger, e.g. heater. Place prone to avoid inhalation of vomit or saliva
2. Loosen clothing round the neck, do not attempt to prise open the mouth as teeth may be broken and inhaled and the tongue pushed back, occluding the airway
3. Give diazepam i.v., 1 + 1mg for each year of life or as rectal preparation, e.g. Stesolid (1–3 years give 5 mg; 10 mg for older children). If no response after 10 minutes give paraldehyde 1 ml for each year of life, in divided dose if more than 2 ml, deep into each buttock. Phenytoin i.v. is an alternative or additional drug if fits continue
4. Continuing seizure/duration longer than 30 minutes is an indication for general anaesthesia. Mechanical ventilation lowers $CO_2$, and should be considered to combat potential cerebral oedema
5. If febrile, undress, tepid sponge, give antipyretic
6. Oral anticonvulsants may be indicated, both short and long term

*Investigations*
Blood glucose (Dextrostix/BM stix), especially during a prolonged fit. Lumbar puncture in first febrile convulsions under 2 years old, prolonged or focal and if meningism present. Others by suspected cause (p 25), e.g. skull and chest X-ray, E and U, serum calcium, Hb and WBC, EEG. A CT scan is indicated in afebrile focal seizures or if focal signs or raised intracranial pressure are present.

*Some types of seizure requiring specific treatment*
1. Infantile spasms: corticosteroids for a course of 4–6 weeks, and a benzodiazepine, e.g. clonazepam
2. Petit mal: ethosuximide or valproate
3. Temporal lobe or focal epilepsy: carbemazepine or valproate, less frequently phenytoin

## Sudden infant death syndrome (SIDS)
*Incidence*
Rate halved from 2 in 1000 to 0.8 in 1000 in Britain. Recent acceleration in fall may be as a result of 'Back to sleep' campaign, placing infants on their backs.

*Definition*
Sudden and unexpected death after which a properly performed autopsy fails to reveal a major cause of death.

*Clinical*
Age 1 month to 1 year old, apparently normal. $\frac{2}{3}$ in winter.
   Maternal smoking increases the risk by a factor of at least two. Overheating implicated, with too much bedding/clothing.
   Failure to appreciate an infant is progressively deteriorating from a relatively minor illness is a factor in some cases.

*Action*
1. Resuscitation may be appropriate
2. If the history and examination do not suggest prior illness or injury and suspicion of the parents seems unfounded, they should be told cot death (SIDS) is likely
3. The Coroner's (Procurator Fiscal in Scotland) duty to investigate is explained together with the need for an autopsy and the role of the police, who will ask for a statement and possibly for identification of the body and may visit the home and remove bedding for examination
4. Emphasis is placed on the routine nature of the inquiries and the absence of a desire to blame parents or the person caring for the victim
5. Parents may wish to hold their baby, and this should be suggested
6. Inform family doctor, health visitor and social services (if involved already)
7. Suppress lactation if breast feeding

## Suspected non-accidental injury (NAI)
Where abuse is or was inflicted or knowingly not prevented by person(s) caring for a child *and* signs are present of physical injury and/or neglect, drug administration, failure to thrive, emotional or sexual abuse.

*Assessment*
1. Injuries inconsistent with explanation, delay in seeking help, medical advice sought for repeated minor injuries
2. Parent young, single, mentally ill, known to social services, low IQ (though remember anyone can be an abusing parent!)
3. Child separated at some time in infancy, child handicapped
4. Physically appears neglected, withdrawn or drugged, bruising of differing ages or bilateral black eyes, scalds or burns, old and new fractures, internal injuries, e.g. subdurals, torn frenulum in mouth, retinal detachment and bleeds, torn abdominal organ, bruising of genitals. If sexual abuse is suspected, a *single* examination is arranged jointly with a Forensic Medical Examiner (specially trained GP usually) and experienced paediatrician to minimize further emotional trauma.

*Investigations*
Photographs, skeletal survey, coagulation studies, venereological/forensic tests.

*Action*
1. Notify senior medical and social work staff immediately
2. Until the child is in a place of safety or security is assured confrontation is best avoided, and then should be undertaken only by experienced staff
3. If removal seems likely seek an Emergency Protection Order (EPO) via social workers or NSPCC. The police do not need a Magistrate's order (useful in an emergency!)
4. Case conference to be called at the earliest possible time to:
    (i) Establish what has taken place: is it NAI?
    (ii) Consider immediate action to protect the child (whether to return home, remain in a place of safety, take out a EPO if not yet obtained, or institute Care Proceedings in the Magistrate's Court)
    (iii) What further information, investigations and procedures may be necessary to make plans for the child's future
    (iv) Should the name of the child, siblings or other children in the household be placed on the 'At risk' register?
    (v) Name a coordinator, the 'key worker', and the 'prime worker', who works with the family (may be the same person)

## MANAGEMENT OF INFANTS SUSPECTED OF INFECTION
1. In the community:
    (i) Most infections are minor, coryzal, and require advice on temperature reduction and an antipyretic. Antibiotic for e.g. pharyngitis, otitis media.
    (ii) Early recognition of the acutely ill infant in the community by parents and family practitioners is an essential first step to bringing the individual for paediatric assessment and reducing morbidity and mortality.

(a) Advise regular observation and temperature taking 4 hourly. Stress that in the neonate a subnormal temperature is of greater significance than fever.
(b) Draw parents' attention to 'sinister' signs being an indication for urgent medical attention, e.g. continuous inconsolable crying for >2 hours, rapid breathing when at rest, seizure, excessive drowsiness, purpuric rash.
(c) If referral to hospital is likely, avoid antibiotics except in the case of suspected meningococcaemia, when penicillin should be given immediately.
2. In the Accident and Emergency Department:
   (i) Sick. Evaluation for focus of infection. If no focus is found, blood culture and urine (clean catch or suprapubic) should be obtained for culture. In an ill infant an LP must be considered. Admit.
   (ii) Pyrexial, no focus clinically, but well enough to go home. Culture as above. Consider broad-spectrum antibiotic, results in lowering the septicaemia rate, without masking possible urinary tract and need for further investigation (p97).

**Suspected infection after foreign travel**
Establish which countries visited and duration there/arrival of a visitor from abroad capable of passing on an illness. Remember, tropical infections often come in twos.
   Infections range from common in UK (e.g. rotavirus, Campylobacter) through unusual (e.g. TB) to rare (e.g. polio, diphtheria), or only from abroad, e.g. rabies, malaria.

1. Fever: from Asia or Africa consider:
   (i) Malaria no matter how long ago the travel and despite taking prophylaxis.
   (ii) Typhoid, hepatitis A (or B if injected, or transfused while abroad), meningococcus. A rash may be present (also consider Dengue haemorrhagic fever virus)
   (iii) TB.
2. Diarrhoea:
   (i) Acute onset: viral commonly, Campylobacter, *E. coli,* dysenteric organisms.
   (ii) Persistent diarrhoea with abdominal pain is suggestive of Giardia lamblia, with mucus ± blood in amoebiasis.
   (iii) Worm infestation is often asymptomatic.
3. Fever + neurological symptoms: polio, falciparum malaria, typhoid, rabies.
4. Fever + sore throat: common infection likely but diphtheria must be remembered.
5. Fever + jaundice: viral hepatitis; with pallor in malaria; varies from 'flu-like symptoms to a shocked state in yellow fever.

# Abbreviations

| | |
|---|---|
| ABO | Refers to the major blood groups A, B and O |
| ALL | Acute lymphoblastic leukaemia |
| ASD | Atrial septal defect |
| CAH | Congenital adrenal hyperplasia |
| CCF | Congestive cardiac failure |
| CPK | Creative phosphokinase |
| D and V | Diarrhoea and vomiting |
| E and U | Electrolytes and urea (in serum or plasma, includes sodium, potassium, chloride, bicarbonate and urea) |
| ECG | Electrocardiogram |
| EEG | Electroencephalogram |
| ELBW | Extremely low birth weight |
| ESR | Erythrocyte sedimentation rate |
| FTT | Failure to thrive |
| G6PD | Glucose-6-phosphate dehydrogenase |
| Hb | Haemoglobin |
| HIV | Human Immunodeficiency virus/aquired immunodeficiency syndrome |
| ITP | Idiopathic thrombocytopenia |
| i.v. | Intravenous |
| JRA | Juvenile rheumatoid arthritis |
| NAI | Non-accidental injury |
| PDA | Patent ductus arteriosus |
| PR | Time interval between beginning of the P wave and the R wave on an electrocardiograph |
| RDS | Respiratory distress syndrome |
| RSV | Respiratory syncitial virus |
| RTA | Renal tubular acidosis |
| SBE | Subacute bacterial endocarditis |
| TB | Tuberculosis |
| TGA | Transposition of the great arteries |
| TORCH | Congenital infections: Toxoplasmosis, other e.g. syphilis Rubella, Cytomegalovirus, Herpes simplex |
| TSH | Thyroid stimulating hormone |
| URTI | Upper respiratory tract infection |

| UTI | Urinary tract infection |
| VLBW | Very low birth weight |
| VSD | Ventricular septal heart defect |
| WBC | White blood cell count |

# Index